Therapy of Lung Metastases

Contributions to Oncology
Beiträge zur Onkologie

Vol. 30

Series Editors
S. Eckhardt, Budapest; *J. H. Holzner,* Wien;
G. A. Nagel, Göttingen

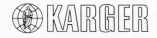

Basel · München · Paris · London · New York · New Delhi · Singapore · Tokyo · Sydney

Proceedings of the Symposium 'Die Therapie von Lungenmetastasen im interdisziplinären Konzept', Heidelberg, June 5th and 6th, 1986

Therapy of Lung Metastases

Volume Editors
P. Drings, I. Vogt-Moykopf, Heidelberg

85 figures and 79 tables, 1988

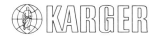

Basel · München · Paris · London · New York · New Delhi · Singapore · Tokyo · Sydney

Contributions to Oncology
Beiträge zur Onkologie

Contents

Contents VI

Preface

The metastasis of a malignant tumor to the lung means its generalization; therefore, the internal therapy of the tumor (chemotherapy and endocrine therapy) stands in the forefront of the therapeutical procedure. However, the results of the last few years and our own experiences show that local treatment (surgical treatment or radiotherapy) in this situation could also be indicated. With internal therapy alone or in combination with other types of treatment there are in many cases good palliative and also potentially curative effects possible.

The Hospital for Thoracic Diseases in Heidelberg-Rohrbach, together with the associations of surgical oncology, medical oncology, pediatric oncology, and radiological oncology of the German Cancer Society as well as with the Tumor Center Heidelberg-Mannheim, arranged a symposium in June 1986 to work out recommendations for the therapy of lung metastases of malignant tumors.

This volume contains the papers presented at this symposium (translated from the original German) and represents an interdisciplinary analysis of current knowledge regarding the treatment of lung metastases. The preconditions, techniques, and results of the surgery of metastases are discussed in detail. For example, it has been found that multiple metastases are no contraindication for surgery if preoperatively it appears possible to remove all visible metastases. The surgical therapy can either follow the chemotherapy to resect the residual metastases or precede it to offer better chances for the chemotherapy because of the reduction of the tumor. The best possible schedule of therapy has to be established in prospective multicentre clinical studies. The results presented in this book and the prognostic factors developed can serve as a basis.

The participants of this symposium came to the conclusion that even in the stage of generalization of a malignant tumor an interdisciplinary approach can be of value for the therapeutical concept.

It is hoped that the reports contained in this volume will offer suggestions for further clinical research on this subject.

Heidelberg, January 1988   *P. Drings,*
                                                        I. Vogt-Moykopf

Biology, Pathology and Diagnosis

Contr. Oncol., vol. 30, pp. 1–16 (Karger, Basel 1988)

Metastasis into the Lung — the Pathologist's Point of View

K. Kayser

Pathology, Hospital for Thoracic Diseases, Heidelberg, FRG

Introduction

It is commonly accepted that malignant tumor growth begins as a local event. The end stage of the disease may again be local. It is, however, a multifocal or generalized disease in the majority of cases. The tumor cells may spread within the regional or distant lymphatic or blood vessels; they may form single or multiple growth centers in a different organ; they may metastasize into various organs or they may spread diffusely all over the whole body. What are the conditions for malignant tumor cells to spread into organs different from the tumor origin? What is the appropriate treatment for a patient suffering from a multifocal tumorous disease? Do metastatic lesions show the same behavior as primary malignancies? Are there morphological aspects of primary tumors and metastases containing some information for the clinicians with respect to prognosis or further treatment?

The ability of tumor cells to metastasize is now understood as a combination of three different phenomena:

(a) It is dependent on the number of malignant cells and, therefore, a stochastic process. Tumor cells have to escape from the bulk tumor and migrate into the lymphatic or blood vessels. Penetration through the basement membrane and invasive activity play a predominant role [27]. Basement membranes act as barriers to the passage of tumor cells [10, 14, 16]. The extracellular matrix has to be degraded by tumor-specific proteases [13, 15].

(b) It is dependent upon the location of the primary tumor in respect to the corresponding organ of metastasis, i.e. a phenomenon of topo-

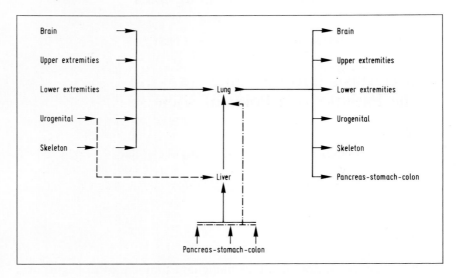

Fig. 1. Scheme of pathways in the process of metastasization.
_____ hematogenous; − · − · − · − lymphogenous-hematogenous;
− − − − per continuitatem, 'serous'.

graphy [2, 25]. The situation is explained in figure 1. The lung and the liver are the central organs for the settlement of metastatic tumor cells escaping from malignancies located in various organs. Both the lung and the liver present a capillary system for filtering tumor cells which may enhance the development of metastases.

(c) The microenvironment plays a predominant role [4, 7, 19, 22]. The ability of tumor cells to grow in an environment different from the primary tumor organ is a prerequisite for metastatic tumor growth. The heterogeneity and different metastatic activity of different lines of tumor cells have experimentally been shown to characterize the metastatic process [3, 6, 18]. Tumor cells have to overcome the local defense mechanisms and − in addition − have to grow faster than the cells of the host. These conditions may explain the fact that solid circumscribed metastases are growing even in organs polluted with tumor cells, and that the diffuse spread of tumor cells is a rare event in human cancer.

Pathologists have analyzed the frequency of metastases in malignant tumors in extensive autopsy studies [1, 30]. These studies are in general of limited value because they present the end stage of a malignant growth in relation to different approaches of treatment, breakdown of the immune system, etc. Examples of the data in these studies are shown in tables I and II. The data of Eder [2] are analyzed for morphology and survival. At the time of death only one metastasis was found in fast-growing tumors, i.e. tumors with short or moderate survival. The majority of these tumors had metastasized into the liver. Tumors accompanied by long survival (5 years or more) showed single metastasis into the lung only in 10–20% of the cases. Especially hypernephromas seem to be a problem for surgical treatment. They show single circumscribed metastases into the lung in 90% of cases. A similar percentage was observed for carcinoma of the colon and of the breast [2].

Table I. Relative frequency of malignant tumors with only 1 metastatic localization at time of death (from Eder, [2])

Primary tumor	Frequency (%)	Key organ	Morphology	Survival rate
Colon	60	liver	homogeneous	medium
Liver	60	lung	homogeneous	medium
Stomach	50	liver	heterogeneous	short
Pancreas	50	liver	heterogeneous	short
Lung	30	–	heterogeneous	short
Kidney	20	lung	homogeneous	long
Mamma	10	lung	homogeneous	long
Prostata	10	lung	homogeneous	long

Table II. Relative frequency of metastases of lung at time of death (from Eder, [2])

Primary tumor	Metastases of lung (%)	Solitary metastases of lung
Colon	31	10
Liver	no data	no data
Stomach	19	12
Pancreas	no data	no data
Kidney	74	60
Mamma	26	10
Prostata	no data	no data
Ovary	20	0

Examination of surgical specimens with metastatic tumors excised for potential curative treatment may be more appropriate in analyzing the dynamic process of malignant growth. It may lead to answers to the following questions:

(a) Do differences exist in the proliferation of tumor cells of metastases compared to tumor cells developed in the host?

(b) Do differences exist in the activation of the immune system of the host tissue between metastatic lesions and tumors of local origin?

(c) How frequent are solid circumscribed metastases compared to multiple metastases?

(d) Do micrometastases exist close to major circumscribed metastases and, if so, what is their clinical significance?

Material and Methods

A detailed macroscopic and microscopic analysis was performed on 31 specimens of intrapulmonary metastases which had migrated from various organs and which were removed during a potentially curative operation. The patients were operated on between Oct. 1, 1985 and March 31, 1986. A list of the material obtained is given in table III. Nineteen patients with metastatic carcinoma and 12 patients with metastatic sarcoma were operated on. Only one major metastasis was found in the majority of the cases. In 4 cases 6 metastases were excised. In 1 case 13 vital metastases were detected (table IV). Additional fibrotic lesions or lung scars probably related to former metastatic lesions were found in 5 cases. The analysis of the vital metastases included metastases from carcinoma of the rectum and testis (8 cases), of the kidneys (3 cases), and of the breast

Table III. Primary Localization of operated intrapulmonary metastases

	n
Sarcomas	12
Carcinomas	19
Testis-Rectum	8
Kidney	3
Mamma	2
Thyroid gland	2
Colon	2
Lung	1
Thymus	1

Table IV. Number of operated intrapulmonary metastases

Metastases (n)	Number of cases			Inactive metastases (n)
	carcinoma	sarcoma	total	
1	8	6	14	2
2	4	2	6	1
3	1	1	2	0
4	1	1	2	1
5	1	0	1	0
6	3	1	4	1
7	0	1	1	0
13	1	0	1	0
Total	19	12	31	5

Table V. Existence of micrometastases close to tumor boundary (< 5 mm)

Micro-metastases	Metastases				Bronchus carcinoma	
	carci-noma	sar-coma	total			
	n	n	n	%	n	%
Existent	4	5	9	29	46	37
Not detectable	15	7	22	71	76	63
Total	19	12	31		122	

(2 cases) (table V). The following parameters were analyzed and graded semi-quantitatively by light microscopy:

(a) Micrometastases near the boundary of the main lesion (less than 0.5 mm),

(b) micrometastases in distant lung parenchyma (> 0.5 mm),

(c) proteolytic activity,

(d) amount of necrotic areas in tumorous lesions,

(e) inflammatory response of host tissue.

The same parameters were examined in surgical specimens of 122 primary bronchus carcinoma for comparison.

Results

Micrometastases

Primary bronchus carcinoma were found to proliferate in bizarre, irregular shapes in the majority of the cases, as shown in a former study [11]. These irregular growth patterns were considered to be partly caused by different growth centers, by the immune response of host tissue, and by the existence of micrometastases at the boundary of the primaries. The proliferation of tumors into the lung tissue seems, therefore, to be connected to multiple implantations of tumor cells near the main lesion. The lung tissue of a complete cross-section of the tumor was screened for micrometastases at a distance of $0-0.5$ mm, and $>0.5-20$ mm. In addition, the excised healthy lung tissue was screened for micrometastases in 3 representative samples. Detected micrometastases of a poorly differentiated epidermoid carcinoma of the lung are

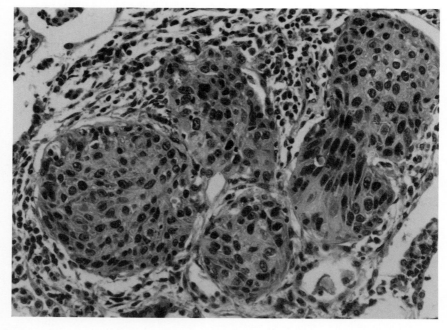

Fig. 2. Micrometastases of a poorly differentiated epidermoid carcinoma (HE, 200:1).

exemplarily shown in figure 2. The frequency of micrometastases was found to decrease with increasing distance. Micrometastases near the boundary of the main tumor ($<$ 0.5 mm) were found in 29% (9/31 cases) in the case of metastatic tumors (table V).

In the case of primary bronchus carcinoma, micrometastases were found in 37% (46/122) of the patients, i.e. in similar percentage. No statistically significant difference between the 'adhesion' of tumor cells originating in primary bronchus carcinoma and metastatic tumors into the lung could be detected. The existence of micrometastases near major tumorous lesions is fairly frequent. Less common are micrometastases at a larger distance from the tumor boundary (table VI). Microimplantations of tumor cells at a distance of 0.5–20 mm measured from the boundary of the main lesion were observed in 11% of primary bronchus carcinoma and in 8% of metastatic tumors into the lung. The frequency of micrometastases located at larger distances is reasonably high. It may be concluded that main tumor lesions are created by agglutination of multiple micrometastases and iterative new implantations of tumor cells near the main lesion due to increased mobility of tumor cells [2, 18, 20]. This theory is in agreement with the predominant role of the microenvironment of the host tissue in influencing tumor growth, and with the observed heterogeneity of the lines of tumor cells [4, 14, 17, 26]. Response to chemoattractants is also reported to be of importance [23, 24, 28]. In the lung this process may be enhanced by the steady movements of the host tissue (breathing) and its empty air spaces.

Table VI. Micrometastases in operated intrapulmonary metastases and in operated primary bronchus carcinoma

Micrometastases	Metastases				Bronchus carcinoma	
	carci-noma	sar-coma	total			
	n	n	n	%	n	%
Existent	2	2	4	8	13	11
Not detectable	17	10	27	92	109	89
Total	19	12	31		122	

Proteolytic Activity

It is commonly accepted that tumor cells need proteolytic enzymes for invasion into blood vessels or into lymphatic vessels [13, 20]. To our knowledge, there is at the moment no technique available measuring proteolytic enzymes in histo-morphologic specimens. However, the preservation of connective lung tissue in the tumorous areas can be considered to be an indicator for activity of proteolytic enzymes of tumor cells. Histo-pathological specimens stained with Sirius H were analyzed for preserved lung parenchyma in the tumorous area and classified as non-detectable, detectable, or complete destruction of connective lung parenchyma in a complete cross section of the metastatic lesion and of the primary bronchus carcinoma. An example of completely preserved interstitial lung tissue in the center of a poorly differentiated epidermoid carcinoma is shown in figure 3.

The results obtained in metastatic tumors and primary bronchus carcinoma are given in table VII. Tumors growing without detectable de-

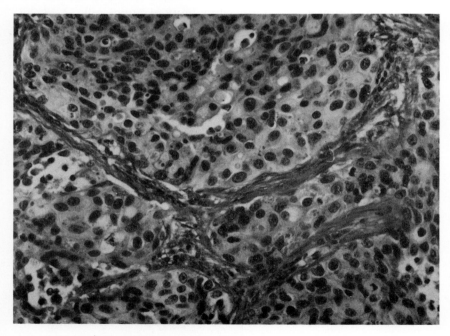

Fig. 3. Completely preserved interstitial lung tissue in the center of a poorly differentiated epidermoid carcinoma (Sirius H, 200:1).

Table VII. Microscopic propagation in specimens of operated intrapulmonary metastases and primary bronchus carcinoma

	Metastases				Bronchus carcinoma	
	carci-noma	sar-coma	total			
	n	n	n	%	n	%
Intra-alveolar	4	0	4	13	27	22
Partially destructive	5	1	6	19	27	22
Totally destructive	10	11	21	68	68	56
Total	19	12	31		122	

struction of interstitial lung tissue were found in 22% (27/122) of the primary bronchus carcinoma and in 20% (4/19) of metastatic carcinoma. Complete destruction of interstitial lung tissue was found in 56% of the bronchus carcinoma (68/122) and in 50% (10/19) of the metastatic carcinoma. Metastatic sarcoma seem to present higher activity of proteolytic enzymes. Eleven out of 12 cases of metastatic sarcoma presented a complete destruction of the original interstitial lung tissue. Metastatic carcinoma into the lung and primary bronchus carcinoma were statistically indistinguishable with respect to these features. They can clearly be separated from metastatic sarcoma into the lung (table VII). The data indicate that degradation of the extracellular matrix is a common property of human malignances, which is in agreement with experimental data [7, 12].

Necrosis

All patients with metastatic lesions into the lung were operated on months or years after excision of the primary tumor followed by post-surgical cytostatic therapy. Especially in cases where sarcomatous lesions were involved, multiple treatments with adjuvant cytostatic therapy were given. Cytostatic therapy was not applied prior to surgery of primary bronchus carcinoma patients. It was expected that necrotic areas in the tumorous lesions should be observed more frequently, and that they should be more extended in metastatic lesions than in primary bronchus carcinoma. The necrotic area was measured in a complete tu-

Table VIII. Number and size of necroses in operated intrapulmonary metastases and operated primary bronchus carcinoma

Necroses	Metastases				. Bronchus carcinoma	
	carci-noma	sar-coma	total			
	n	n	n	%	n	%
None	7	5	12	39	17	14
Slight	5	3	8	26	36	30
Moderate	1	2	3	9	30	24
Extensive	6	2	8	26	39	32
Total	19	12	31		122	

mor cross-section of metastatic lesions and of primary bronchus carcinoma specimens. The cases were grouped as follows (necrotic/tumor area): no necrosis — slight necrosis (20%) — moderate necrosis (20% – 70%) — extensive necrosis (> 70%).

The results of our analysis are given in table VIII. The findings were contrary to our expectations.

No to minimum necrotic areas were found in 39% (12/31) of the metastatic lesions and only in 14% (17/122) of the primary bronchus carcinomas. Severe necrotic lesions covering more than 70% of a complete cross-section were found in 26% of the metastatic lesions (8/31) and in 32% (39/122) of the primary bronchus carcinoma. The data may be interpreted as showing that an important percentage of metastatic lesions do not respond to chemotherapy and that excision of these lesions is a necessity from the therapeutic point of view. Necrotic areas in primary bronchus carcinomas are fairly common.

Inflammatory Response

Inflammatory response of host tissue due to growth of the primary bronchus carcinoma is observed frequently [9]. In the majority of cases it is related to a cell-mediated host reaction of the lung tissue [12]. The dominant subpopulation of the inflammatory cells was found to be T cells [5, 12, 31]. The relation of T-helper/suppressor cells was measured as 1.8 : 1 at the boundary of bronchus carcinoma, i.e. in a relation

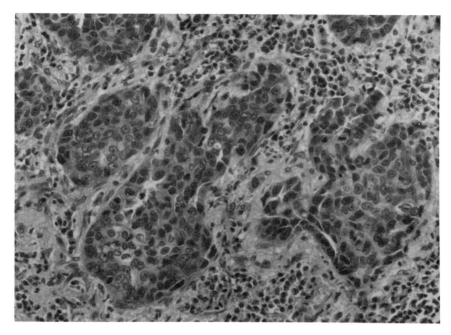

Fig. 4. Dense inflammatory response of host tissue at the boundary of a poorly differentiated adenocarcinoma (HE, 200 : 1).

similar to that observed in the peripheral blood [12]. The existence of dense inflammatory infiltrations at the boundary of a poorly differentiated adenocarcinoma of the lung is exemplarily shown in figure 4. The number of lymphocytes was measured at the boundary of metastatic lesions and of the primary bronchus carcinoma in paraffin-embedded, HE-stained specimens; they were grouped as follows:

Scattered lymphocytes: 50 lymphocytes/unit area (0.04 mm^2)

Dense lymphocytes: > 50 lymphocytes/unit area (0.04 mm^2).

Inflammatory response of host tissue due to growth of the primary bronchus carcinoma was observed in 43% (53/122). In the case of metastatic lesions only one tumor was found with moderate to severe inflammatory infiltrations at the tumor boundary. In nearly all cases of metastatic tumors no inflammatory response of host tissue could be observed. For a correct interpretation of these data the tumor volume has to be taken into account. Inflammatory response of host tissue increases

Table IX. Inflammatory response in operated intrapulmonary metastases and primary bronchus carcinoma

Inflammation	Metastases				Bronchus carcinoma	
	carci-noma	sar-coma	total			
	n	n	n	%	n	%
None − minimal	18	12	30	97	69	57
Moderate − severe	1	0	1	3	53	43
Total	19	12	31		122	

with increasing tumor volume, with the exception of tumor volume between 40 cm³ and 60 cm³ where a decline has been observed [11]. The tumor volume of the primary carcinoma of the lung and of the metastatic lesions into the lung is shown in table IX. Primary bronchus carcinomas have a tumor volume 32.1 ± 5.4 cm³ at the time of excision. No statistically significant differences between the different cell types were found. Metastatic lesions at the time of operation were considerably larger. Metastatic sarcomas measured 234 ± 12 cm³, i.e. they present a tumor mass which is not eligible for curative surgical treatment in most patients suffering from primary bronchus carcinoma. Primary bronchus carcinomas measuring 100 cm³ or more are accompanied by an inflammatory response of host tissue in nearly 100% of cases [11]. The complete lack of inflammatory response in the case of metastatic lesions into the lung (except in 1 case) is, therefore, not related to the tumor volume. It is probably an expression of different biological behavior towards metastatic tumor growth in respect to the 'activation' of the immune system of the host tissue. It seems fair to conclude that, in contrast to the reaction to primary bronchus carcinomas, recognition of metastatic tumorous growth is not possible by the immune system of the host.

Excised Lung Tissue

As a rule, primary bronchus carcinomas are excised including the complete tumor-bearing lobe or lung [29]. Metastatic lesions are generally excised by extended wedge excision [29]. The tumor volume of the metastatic lesions and of the primary lung carcinoma was measured as follows: The resection specimens were insufflated by buffered formalin (7%) via the main bronchus and simultaneously expanded by insufflation of air of moderate pressure (50 mm Hg). The specimens were allowed to fix for an additional 24 h, and were then cut into slices 6 mm thick. The tumor area of each lung slice was measured using a graphic pad. The total volume of the tumor was measured by adding the tumor area of each lung slice multiplied by its thickness. The mean tumor volume was calculated after logarithmic transformation of the original data. The mean tumor volume of metastases and primary bronchus carcinomas is shown in table X. The relation between excised healthy lung volume and tumor volume in the case of metastatic lesions and in the

Table X. Tumor size of surgically excised intrapulmonary metastases and primary bronchus carcinoma

	n	Tumor volume (cm^3) (confidence limits > 0.95)
Bronchus carcinoma	122	32.1 ± 5.4
Epidermoid	56	27.5 ± 4
Adeno	27	38.8 ± 9
Large cell	13	35.5 ± 12
Small cell	12	35.9 ± 12
Metastases		
Carcinoma	31	133.0 ± 63
Sarcoma	19	70.0 ± 32
Lung parenchyma	31	322.0 ± 180

Table XI. Tumor mass and surgically excised lung parenchyma

	n	Volume (cm^3)		Relation tumor-lung
		tumor	lung parenchyma	
Metastases	31	133	322	0.41
Bronchus carcinoma	122	32	640	0.05

case of primary bronchus carcinomas is shown in table XI. Primary bronchus carcinomas occupied only 5% of excised lung tissue. In the case of metastatic lesions this percentage rose to 41%. The relation between excised tumor volume and additionally removed healthy lung tissue is acceptable even in the case of a palliative operation of metastatic lesions. Excision of malignant primaries with potential curative treatment is only possible taking into account a large amount of excised healthy lung tissue compared to tumorous tissue.

Conclusion

The biological behavior of malignant primaries leading to metastatic lesions into the lung is not yet completely understood. Analysis of resection specimens containing metastatic tumors into the lung and containing primary bronchus carcinomas led to two major conclusions:

(a) The absence of inflammatory infiltrations at the boundary of metastatic lesions is to be interpreted as inactivity of the immune system of the host tissue (i.e. no detectable immune response).

(b) There is an indication of increased activity of proteolytic enzymes in the case of metastatic sarcoma into the lung.

Both observations are in agreement with results obtained from animal experiments. Proteolytic activity was found to be a necessity for metastasis in experimental tumor models. Schirrmacher [21] reported a strong decline in metastatic potential in experimental tumor models after enhancement of the cell-mediated immune response of host tissue. The propagation of tumor growth into the lung tissue is similar for metastatic tumors and for primary lung carcinomas. The host tissue influences tumor propagation to some extent. The implantation of micrometastases near the main metastasis is fairly common in metastatic and primary lung tumors. The main lesion can be understood as an agglutination of multiple micrometastases. This fact may explain the existence of solid circumscribed metastases in liver and lung enhanced by the texture properties of these organs.

Surgical treatment of tumor metastases into the lung should be considered with regard to the amount of healthy lung tissue to be excised. Excision of primary malignancies of the lung with potentially curative treatment is generally performed by additional extensive excision of healthy lung tissue – only 5% of excised lung tissue is actually destroyed by tumor cells. Excision of metastatic tumors can be performed while removing a smaller amount of healthy lung tissue: on average, 41% of excised tissue has been destroyed by tumor cells. In addition to other well-known medical considerations, these different percentages should be taken into account when ethical problems of adjuvant tumor surgery are being discussed.

References

1 Abrams, H. L.; Spiro, R.; Goldstein, N.: Metastases in carcinoma. Analysis of 1000 autopsied cases. Cancer *3:* 74–81 (1950).

2 Eder, M.: Die Metastasierung: Fakten und Probleme aus humanpathologischer Sicht. Verh. dt. Ges. Path. *68:* 1–11 (1984).

3 Fidler, I. J.: Selection of successive tumor lines for metastasis. Nature new Biol. *242:* 148–149 (1973).

4 Fidler, I. J.; Nicolson, G. L.: Brief communication: Organ selectivity for implantation, survival, and growth of B 16 melanoma variant tumor lines. J. natn. Cancer Inst. *57:* 1199–1202 (1976).

5 Furukawa, T.; Watanabe, S.; Kodama, T. et al.: T-Zone histiocytes in adenocarcinoma of the lung in relation to postoperative prognosis. Cancer *56:* 2651–2656 (1985).

6 Hart, I. R.; Fidler, I. J.: The implication of tumor heterogeneity for studies on the biology and therapy of cancer metastasis. Biochem. biophys. Acta *651:* 37–50 (1981).

7 Hart, I. R.: "Seed and soil" revisited: Mechanisms of site specific metastasis. Cancer Met. Rev. *42:* 331–341 (1982).

8 Hujanen, E. S.; Terranova, V. P.: Migration of tumor cells to organ-derived chemoatractants. Cancer Res. *45:* 3517–3521 (1985).

9 Ioachim, H. L.; Dorsett, B. L.; Paluch, E.: The immune response at the tumor site in lung carcinoma. Cancer *38:* 2296–2309 (1976).

10 Jones, P. A.; DeClerck, Y. A.: Destruction of extracellular matrix containing glycoproteins, elastin, and collagen by metastatic tumor cells. Cancer Res. *40:* 3222–3227 (1980).

11 Kayser, K.; Ebert, W.; Merkle, N. M.; Becker, H. D.: Defense mchanism and macroscopic tumor growth in lung tissue. J Cancer Res. Clin. Oncol. *111:* 277–283 (1986).

12 Kayser, K.; Bülzebruck, H.; Ebert, W. et al.: Local tumor inflammation, lymph node metastasis and survival of operated bronchus carcinoma patients. J. natn. Cancer Inst. *77:* 77–81 (1986).

13 Kramer, R. H.; Nicolson, G. L.: Invasion of vascular endothelial cell monolayers and underlying matrix by metastatic human cancer cells; in Schweiger, International cell biology, pp. 194–199 (Springer, Berlin, Heidelberg, New York, Tokyo 1981).

14 Liotta, L. A.; Kleinermann, J.; Catanzaro, P.: Degradation to basement membrane by murine tumor cells. J. Natn. Cancer Inst. *58:* 1427–1431 (1977).

15 Liotta, L. A.; Abe, S.; Gehron-Robey, P.: Preferential digestion of basement membrane collagen by an enzyme derived from a metastatic murine tumor. Proc. Natn. Acad. Sci. USA 76: 2268–2272 (1979).

16 Liotta, L. A.: Tumor invasion and metastases: Role of the basement membrane. Am. J. Path. 117: 339–348 (1984).

17 Suzuki, M.; Hori, K.; Abe, I. et al.: Functional characterization of the microcirculation in tumors. Cancer Met. Rev. 3: 115–126 (1984).

18 Nicolson, G. L.; Custead, S. E.: Tumor metastasis is not due to adaptation of cells to new organ environment. Science 215: 176–178 (1982).

19 Nicolson, G. L.; Poste, G.: Tumor cell diversity and host responses in cancer metastasis: Part I. Properties of metastatic cells. Curr. Probl. Cancer 6: 1–83 (1982).

20 Nicolson, G. L.: Generation of phenotypic diversity and progression in metastatic tumor cells. Cancer Met. Rev. 3: 25–42 (1984).

21 Schirrmacher, V.: Eigenschaften von Tumorzellen als Voraussetzung der Metastasierung: Untersuchungen zum metastatischen Phänotyp. Verh. Dt. Ges. Path. 68: 12–17 (1984).

22 Shearman, P. J.; Longenecker, B. M.: Clonal variation and functional correlation of organ-specific metastasis-associated antigen. Int. J. Cancer 27: 387–395 (1981).

23 Sträuli, P.; Weiss, L.: Cell locomotion and tumour penetration. Report on a workshop of the EORTC cell surface project group. Eur. J. Cancer 13: 1–12 (1977).

24 Sträuli, P.; Haemmerli, G.: The role of cancer cell motility in invasion. Cancer Met. Rev. 3: 127–141 (1984).

25 Sugarbaker, E. V.: Patterns of metastasis in human malignancies. Cancer Biol. Rev. 2: 235–278 (1981).

26 Talmadge, J. E.: The selective nature of metastasis. Cancer Met. Rev. 2: 25–40 (1983).

27 Terranova, V. P.; Hujanen, E. S.; Martin, G. R.: Basement membrane and the invasive activity of metastatic tumor cells. J. Natn. Cancer Inst. 77: 311–316 (1986).

28 Varani, J.; Fligiel, S. E.; Perone, P.: Directed motility in strongly malignant murine tumor cells. Int. J. Cancer 35: 559–561 (1985).

29 Vogt-Moykopf, I.; Toomes, H.; Heinrich, S.: Sleeve resection of the bronchus and pulmonary artery for pulmonary lesions. Thorac. cardiovasc. Surg. 31: 193–198 (1983).

30 Walther, H. E.: Krebsmetastasen (Schwabe, Basel, 1948).

31 Watanabe, S.; Sato, Y.; Kodama, T.: Immuno-histochemical study with monoclonal antibodies on immune response in human lung cancers. Cancer Res. 43: 5883–5889 (1983).

Prof. Dr.-med. K. Kayser, Abteilung Pathologie, Krankenhaus Rohrbach,
Klinik für Thoraxerkrankungen der LVA Baden,
Amalienstr. 5, D-6900 Heidelberg (FRG)

Contr. Oncol., vol. 30, pp. 17−27 (Karger, Basel 1988)

New Experimental Approaches to the Therapy of Metastasis in Tumor Model Systems

V. Schirrmacher

Institut für Immunologie und Genetik, Deutsches Krebsforschungszentrum, Heidelberg, FRG

I would like to review our experience with the application of non-oncogenic viruses for cancer therapy in metastasizing tumor model systems. The rationale has been to use viruses to modify tumor cell surfaces and thereby activate and direct immune responses against tumor cells which have been successfully selected through evolution for protection against infectious diseases. Such responses include activation of lymphokines, of natural defence reactions and of specific immune responses. In our search for effective anti-metastatic therapy protocols we have used and tested different viruses and concepts, including oncolysis and xenogenization. The tumor models were of murine or human origin. One model was the highly metastatic murine lymphosarcoma ESb [19] which affects multiple visceral organs. The other is a malignant human melanoma (MeWo) growing in immunodeficient nude mice, a tumor system which has recently been introduced as a model of human cancer metastasis [12].

The Eb/ESb Mouse Tumor Model System

Most of the experiments in this study were performed with the mouse tumor ESb, which is a spontaneous, highly metastatic variant of the methylcholanthrene-induced T cell lymphoma L 5178 YE (Eb) [19, 21]. According to our recent analysis, this spontaneous variant most likely arose by fusion of the original lymphoma with a host macrophage, a process which was followed by chromosome segregation and rearrangements [14]. The variant expresses cell surface markers of T cells and macrophages [15], is highly invasive in organ culture systems [23], can penetrate blood vessel endothelium and sub-endothelial extra-cellular matrix in vitro [26] and expresses and secretes several degradative enzymes [13, 27]. When transplanted subcutaneously into normal syngeneic DBA/2 mice, fewer than 10 cells of this tumor line can grow, metastasize and kill the host within a few weeks. Because of the aggressiveness of the tumor and the speed with which it infiltrates internal organs, in particular liver, spleen and lung [19], this tumor is very difficult to treat. Because of this toughness we consider this tumor a challenge for the design of effective anti-metastatic therapy strategies. In this model we have tested different treatment procedures such as surgery, chemotherapy, unspecific immune stimulation [25] and adoptive immune cell transfer [18, 21]. We were interested in comparing the relative efficiency of different treatment procedures to prevent outgrowth of metastases, thereby prolonging life or eradicating metastases and thus curing the animal of its disease.

Tumor Antigen Expression and Immune Escape of ESb Cells

This ESb tumor model was found to be amenable to immunological intervention. We have characterized on this tumor a tumor-associated transplantation antigen (TATA) which can induce weak protective immunity [4] and which can activate specific cytotoxic T lymphocytes (CTL) [20]. Good therapeutic effects were achieved by adoptive transfer of immune T cells directed against the TATA [21] and also by immune T cells directed against minor histocompatibility antigens [18].

One problem with specific immunotherapy protocols in this model, however, has been the generation of specific immune escape variants. This problem could not be overcome by using homogeneous cloned tumor antigen-positive cell lines. We found that during metastasis of such cells from a subcutaneous inoculation site, after about 12 days immune escape variants developed in the spleen [5, 6]. Such variants were specifically immuno-resistant to lysis by anti-tumor CTL. Recently we have made progress in the understanding of basic mechanisms underlying the generation of such immune escape variants. The variants do not change the expression of the H-2K^d restricting molecules [1] but change the expression of the TATA so that they cannot be recognized by corresponding CTLs. Such variants were found to arise with a high frequency even in animals which were specifically preimmunized against ESb cells [6]. This might explain the relative inefficiency of specific immunization procedures involving high doses of irradiated tumor cells [4]. Recently we were able to induce reexpression of the tumor antigen in such immune escape variants [3]. We conclude from these experiments that the variants represent gene regulatory variants rather than true mutants.

In the meantime, we have found ways to overcome − at least partially − the problem of the generation of immune escape variants. The immunogenicity of this tumor was found to depend very much on the site of inoculation. The best immunogenicity was obtained with viable tumor cells inoculated into the pinna. By following this inoculation procedure a stronger tumor-specific immune response was evoked than in the case of s.c. or i.p. inoculations, and occasionally we even observed spontaneous tumor regressions in such animals. In addition, we have established procedures of increasing the tumor cells' immunogenicity by the introduction of additional new antigens into the tumor cell surface, via mutagenization [2] or infection by viruses [10].

Application of Viruses for Tumor Xenogenization and Oncolysis

Particularly impressive therapeutic effects were seen with the latter approach when we applied myxoviruses for cancer therapy. We used both lytic and non-lytic myxoviruses such as influenza A (Flu) or Newcastle Disease Virus (NDV). These viruses can bind to the tumor cell surface, infect the cells and replicate therein, thereby expressing viral antigens on the cell surface. The cell surface is also the site where the maturing viruses are budding. The lytic virus strains destroy the infected target cells and reinfect neighboring cells, while the nonlytic strains do not destroy the infected target cells and do not reinfect neighboring cells. While lytic viruses can have direct anti-tumor effects (oncolysis), non-lytic viruses can have indirect anti-tumor effects by stimulating host immune responses and by increasing the tumor cell's immunogenicity (xenogenization). Tumor therapeutic effects were observed with myxoviruses in both the mouse and the human metastatic tumor model system. To understand differences between lytic and non-lytic viruses it is important to understand their mode of infection and replication. Infection of a cell by a virus is initiated by adsorption, i.e. the attachment of the virus particles to the cell surface. Following this step, NDV and

Flu seem to differ in their mechanism of cell penetration. While influenza viruses infect cells mainly via a pinocytotic process, penetration of NDV results mainly from the fusion of the viral envelope with the host cell membrane via a specialized fusion protein. The avirulent substrain Ulster, when harvested from the allantoic fluid of embryonated eggs, can infect a variety of cells and replicate in them (monocyclic replication). The virus produced by infected cells, however, has no active fusion protein and therefore cannot spread and infect other cells. The inactive fusion protein, however, can be activated by proteolytic cleavage. While influenza viruses have a broad host range, NDV, isolated from chicken, has a rather limited host range.

In comparison with influenza virus, NDV is a much less hazardous virus for man and therefore has the potential for clinical application. Its use as an antineoplastic agent was proposed, because of its low neurotropism, as early as 1965 [7]. Oncolysates of NDV infected human tumor cells have already been applied quite successfully in the clinic for postsurgical management of stage II malignant melanoma [8]. During a long observation period of clinical application in cancer patients, even lytic strains of NDV did not cause side-effects (W. Cassel, personal communication). Another important aspect is the strong potency of NDV to induce interferon in different species including man [11, 16] and thus to stimulate natural defence mechanisms [9].

Oncolysis by Means of Lytic Virus Strains

Following the classical studies of Lindenmann, who used the virulent strain M-tur of influenza A virus (Flu) for therapy studies of nonmetastatic transplantation tumors, we tested this virus for therapeutic effects using the highly metastatic tumor ESb. Details of these experiments are described elsewhere [24]. (DBA/2 × A2G) F-1 animals were inoculated with 10^5 ESb cells i.p., and 6 days later, when ascites cells were growing out, one inoculation of virus was given i.p. to induce an oncolytic effect in the peritoneum. At optimal virus dosages ($2 \times 10^4 - 5 \times 10^4$ TCIU) we observed more than 100% life prolongation of all the treated animals, and about 20–30% of the animals survived. These therapeutic results were particularly remarkable compared to the effects of chemotherapy obtained with antimetastatic drugs, where we observed less life prolongation and no cures.

Next we investigated the therapeutic effects of viral oncolysis by using the lytic myxoviruses NDV (Italian) or influenza A in the human tumor model (MeWo grown in nude mice) [12]. We first isolated a metastatic subline, MeWo-Met, as described in [24].

The therapy experiments [24] were performed with this MeWo-Met line, which was transplanted into Balb/c (nu/nu) mice in the form of in vitro-invaded brain tissue aggregates. After the tumors had taken, we started a therapy with oncolytic virus. Because of the pathogenicity of influenza A virus to these immunodeficient mice, we changed to a less pathogenic virus and used the Italien strain of Newcastle Disease Virus (NDV). We first made sure that this virulent strain could be tolerated by the nude mice. Tumor therapy with NDV (Italian) was started after about 1 month when the locally growing MeWo tumor was readily visible. Control animals received inoculations of allantoic fluid which was free of virus. The virus or the control fluid was inoculated directly into the tumor by means of multiple inoculations and also intravenously and subcutaneously. Altogether, the animals were treated 4 times. It was found that the growth of the highly malignant tumor melanoma line was stopped in the group treated with the lytic NDV strain. By contrast, in the control groups there was a continuous and steady tumor growth, so that the tumor became very large and multinodular with certain areas becoming necrotic and others growing progressively. At the end of the experiment the animals were killed and investigated histologically. The results indicated that the virus treatment which had profoundly affected the local tumor growth had not significantly affected the metastases of this tumor.

In conclusion, we were able to establish a human melanoma tumor line in nude mice (MeWo-Met) which can metastasize to lung, liver and spleen. Furthermore, we could show profound therapeutic effects following inoculations of the locally growing tumors by oncolytic NDV strains. We could not, however, achieve therapeutic effects upon MeWo-Met metastases. It is likely that the virus was not able to reach the metastases. It has to be kept in mind that the possibility of generating systemic T cell mediated anti-tumor immunity following virus infection of the tumor cells was excluded by the use of athymic nude mice. We will show below, however, that in immunocompetent mice systemic anti-metastatic effects can be obtained with the help of NDV when using appropriate protocols.

Xenogenization by Means of Non-Lytic Virus

Human Tumor Model (WeWo)

We reported above that highly malignant human melanoma cells growing in nude mice could be successfully treated by direct inoculation of a virulent lytic strain of NDV. No such effects were observed when using the non-lytic strain Ulster. We think that one reason for the difference in effectiveness of lytic as compared to non-lytic virus in this system was perhaps the different ability to spread to neighboring cells.

To circumvent the problem of unequal distribution of virus within the tumor we designed a different type of experiment and tested the effect of admixture of virus-infected tumor cells to non-infected cells. In the control group we inoculated 5 million MeWo-Met cells subcutaneously. After a lag phase of about 3 weeks primary tumors could be seen and they continued growing progressively for about 2 months until the animals died. In the second group where we admixed 1 million NDV (Ulster)-infected MeWo-Met cells to 5 million non-infected MeWo-Met cells, we saw a very dramatic retardation in the outgrowth of the primary tumor [24]. The lag phase before tumor take was delayed and the growth rate of the tumor was significantly decreased when compared to the control. So far we know very little about the underlying mechanisms of this tumor suppression by 20% virus-infected human tumor cells. Since the effect was observed in nude mice and the virus was a non-lytic virus, it is likely that the effect was due to an activation of natural defense mechanisms. Such mechanisms have been studied by Reid et al. [17] and were attributed to interferon production and NK cell cytotoxicity.

Mouse Tumor Model (ESb)

We described above that lytic virus inoculated directly into a growing ESb ascites tumor could have rather striking therapeutic effects. We also investigated the effect of non-lytic virus in syngeneic animals in which ESb tumors were growing subcutaneously. Successive inoculations of NDV (Ulster) into such growing tumors every second day led to local tumor regression and to survival of about 40% of the treated animals, while in the control groups all animals died from outgrowth of metastases [24]. In parallel we have used an immune escape variant from the same tumor which does not express tumor antigens sufficient for immune recognition. None of the animals inoculated with this tumor variant could be successfully treated with NDV Ulster when using the same protocol as above. These results thus clearly indicate that a therapeutic effect of direct inoculation of nonlytic virus into a locally growing tumor depends on immune recognition of a specific tumor antigen.

Postoperative Immunotherapy in the ESb Model with Virally Modified Tumor Cells

Having seen the direct anti-tumor effects of NDV-Ulster inoculation into a locally growing ESb tumor, we next tested the applicability to anti-metastatic therapy. We were interested in testing whether NDV-modified tumor cells could be used in tumor-bearing animals, in which the primary tumor had been operated on, to prevent the outgrowth of metastases. The postoperative immunotherapy protocol was as follows: DBA/2 animals were inoculated with 5×10^4 ESb tumor cells intradermally in the back and operated on when the tumor was still small (5 – 7 mm diameter). Removal of the primary tumor at this time was not curative because the animals had already developed micrometastases which led to death within about 3 weeks. As described in detail elsewhere [10], we observed good therapeutic effects when using for postoperative immunotherapy NDV-modified irradiated ESb tumor cells. About 50% of such treated animals became long-term survivors and developed specific long-lasting anti-tumor immunity [22]. In contrast, post-operative immunization with irradiated ESb tumor cells alone was totally ineffective. Since the survivors of the postoperative immunotherapy with ESb-NDV developed long-lasting anti-tumor immunity, the therapy appeared to have widespread systemic effects.

Investigations into the mechanism of this anti-metastatic therapy revealed the following information:

1. The therapeutic effect depended on the presence of mature T lymphocytes.

2. The therapeutic effect depended on the presence of a tumor antigen.

3. Optimal therapeutic effects required direct contact of virus and tumor cells.

4. Therapeutic effects were observed with low doses of virus while higher doses were less or non-efficient.

In vitro analyses of anti-tumor immune responses were performed to investigate the effect of viral modification on the immune response.

The frequency of tumor specific cytotoxic T lymphocyte precursor cells (CTLP) with specificity for the ESb tumor was about 1 in 15,000 in spleens of ESb immune animals, while it was 1 in about 6,500 cells in ESb-NDV immune animals. This increase in CTLP frequency is markable, because the limiting dilution analysis was performed in the presence of excess Il-2 so that helper cells were not required. When testing the tumor specific CTL response in bulk cultures we again observed an increased response. The highest cytotoxicity was seen when NDV-infected ESb cells were used both for priming in vivo and for restimulation in vitro [28].

In figure 1 we have summarized the crucial points in our concept of immunotherapy of micrometastases. At the time of therapy, the mouse carries the primary tumor (P) and the micrometastases in internal organs such as the spleen (S), as well as immune T cells (cytolytic T lymphocyte precursors, CTLP) sensitized against the tumor antigen of ESb cells. We anticipate co-existence at this time of immune cells and tumor cells not only in the spleen but also in the blood and perhaps in other organs. From our in vitro analysis it appears that the immune T cells are not activated and need further signals to become overtly cytotoxic. Our concept for immunotherapy consists of: (1) reduction of tumor burden by surgery, and (2) post-operative immunization with a vaccine

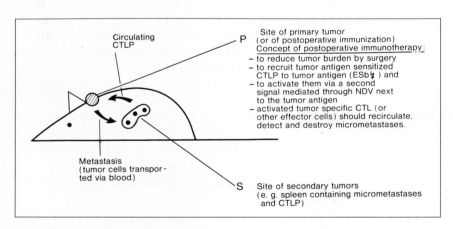

Fig. 1. Concept of postoperative immunotherapy of metastases in the ESb tumor model of the mouse. CTLP = cytolytic T lymphocyte precursors; CTC = cytolytic T lymphocytes.

containing the corresponding tumor antigen and an agent that might function as a second signal. We believe that NDV can mediate this second signal in conjunction with the tumor antigen. The immunogen is inoculated at different sites around the removed primary tumor and might there recruit from the circulation the sensitized CTLP which then recognize the tumor antigen in the vaccine. Upon this interaction, the CTLP might receive a second signal for activation mediated through NDV. Such a cytotoxicity-amplifying effect has been observed both in vitro and in vivo and it might involve interferons. Following this activation in the periphery, activated tumor-specific CTL or other immune effector T cells similarly activated might recirculate and be able to detect and destroy micrometastases in internal organs, especially those in the liver and spleen which are the predominant sites of metastasis in this tumor model.

Acknowledgements

I would like to thank my collaborators, R. Heicappell, P. von Hoegen, T. Ahlert and B. Appelhans, for their invaluable contributions, and A. Griesbach for help with the animal experiments. The excellent typing assistance of Mrs. Heidrun Zimmermann is gratefully acknowledged.

References

1 Altevogt, P.; Leidig, S.; Heckl-Östreicher, B.: Resistance of metastatic tumor variants to tumor-specific cytotoxic T-lymphocytes not due to defects in expression of restricting major histocompatibility complex molecules in murine cells. Cancer Res. *44:* 5305–5313 (1984).

2 Altevogt, P.; Hoegen, P. von; Leidig, S.; Schirrmacher, V.: Effects of mutagens on the immunogenicity of tumor cells: immunological and biochemical evidence for altered cell surface antigens. Cancer Res. *45:* 4270–4277 (1985).

3 Altevogt, P.; Hoegen, P. von; Schirrmacher, V.: Immunoresistant metastatic tumor variants can reexpress their tumor antigen by treatment with agents that inhibit DNA-methylation. Int. J. Cancer (in press).

4 Bosslet, K.; Schirrmacher, V.; Shantz, G.: Tumor metastases and cell-mediated immunity in a model system in DBA/2 mice. VI. Similar specificity patterns of protective anti-tumor immunity in vivo. Int. J. Cancer *24:* 303–313 (1979).

5 Bosslet, K.; Schirrmacher, V.: Escape of metastasizing clonal tumor cell variants from tumor-specific cytolytic T lymphocytes. J. exp. Med. *154:* 557–561 (1981).

6   Bosslet, K.; Schirrmacher, V.: High-frequency generation of new immunoresistant
    tumor variants during metastasis of a cloned murine tumor line (ESb). Int. J. Can-
    cer *29:* 195–202 (1982).

7   Cassel, W. A.; Garret, R. E.: Newcastle Disease Virus as an anti-neoplastic agent.
    Cancer *18:* 863–868 (1965).

8   Cassel, W. A.; Murray, D. R.; Phillips, H. S.: A phase II study on the postsurgical
    management of stage II malignant melanoma with a Newcastle Disease Virus onco-
    lysate. Cancer *52:* 856–860 (1983).

9   Hamburg, S. I.; Cassell, G. H.; Rabinovich, M.: Relationship between enhanced
    macrophage phagocytic activity and the induction of interferon by Newcastle Dis-
    ease virus in mice. J. Immun. 1360–1364 (1980).

10 Heicappell, R.; Schirrmacher, V.; Hoegen, P. von et al.: Prevention of metastatic
    spread by postoperative immunotherapy with virally modified autologous tumor
    cells. Int. J. Cancer *37:* 569–577 (1986).

11 Ito, Y.; Nagai, Y.; Maeno, K.: Interferon production in mouse spleen cells and
    mouse fibroblasts (L cells) stimulated by various strains of Newcastle Disease virus.
    J. gen. Virol. *62:* 349–352 (1982).

12 Kerbel, R. S.; Man, M. S.; Dexter, D.: A model of human cancer metastasis: exten-
    sive spontaneous and artificial metastasis of a human pigmented melanoma and
    derived variant sublines in nude mice. J. Natn. Cancer Inst. *72:* 93–108 (1984).

13 Kramer, M. D.; Robinson, P.; Vlodavsky, I. et al.: Characterization of an extracellu-
    lar matrix-degrading protease derived from a highly metastatic tumor cell line.
    Eur. J. Cancer Clin. Oncol. *21:* 307–316 (1985).

14 Larizza, L.; Schirrmacher, V.; Pflüger, E.: Acquisition of high metastatic capacity
    after in vitro fusion of a non-metastatic tumor line with a bone-marrow derived
    macrophage. J. exp. Med. *160:* 1579–1584 (1984).

15 Larizza, L.; Schirrmacher, V.; Graf, L. et al.: Suggestive evidence that the highly
    metastatic variant ESb of the T cell lymphoma Eb is derived from spontaneous fu-
    sion with a host macrophage. Int. J. Cancer *34:* 699–707 (1984).

16 Merigan, T. C.; De Clergu, E.; Findelstein, M. S. et al.: Clinical studies employing
    interferon inducers in man and animals. Ann. N.Y. Acad. Sci. *173:* 746–759 (1970).

17 Reid, L. M.; Minato, N.; Jones, C. et al.: Rejection of virus persistently infected tu-
    mor cells and its implications for regulation of tumor growth and metastasis in
    athymic nude mice; in Reed, Proc. 3rd Int. Workshop On Nude Mice, Montana
    State University, Bozeman, Montana, 1979, vol. 2, pp. 505–526 (Gustav Fischer,
    New York 1982).

18 Schirrmacher, V.: Tumor metastases and cell-mediated immunity in a model system
    in DBA/2 mice. V. Transfer of protective immunity with H-2 identical immune T
    cells from B10.D2 mice. Int. J. Cancer *24:* 80–86 (1979).

19 Schirrmacher, V.; Shantz, G.; Clauer, K. et al.: Tumor metastases and cell-mediated
    immunity in a model system in DBA/2 mice. I. Tumor invasiveness in vitro and
    metastases formation in vivo. Int. J. Cancer *23:* 233–244 (1979).

20 Schirrmacher, V.; Bosslet, K.; Shantz, G. et al.: Tumor metastases and cell-mediated
    immunity in a model system in DBA/2 mice. IV. Antigenic differences between the
    parental tumor line and its metastasizing variant. Int. J. Cancer *23:* 245–252
    (1979).

21 Schirrmacher, V.; Fogel, M.; Russmann, E. et al.: Antigenic variation in cancer

metastasis. Immune escape versus immune control. Cancer Met. Rev. *1:* 241–274 (1982).

22   Schirrmacher, V.; Heicappell, R.: Prevention of metastatic spread by postoperative immunotherapy with virally modified autologous tumor cells. II. Establishment of specific systemic anti tumor immunity. Clin. exp. Met. *5:* 147–159 (1987).

23   Schirrmacher, V.; Braun, M.; Waller, C. A. et al.: Changes in adhesive, invasive and metastatic capacity of a T lymphoma after fusion with a bone marrow derived macrophage; in Macher, Sorg, Local immunity in cancer, pp. 72–83 (Regensburg & Biermann, Münster 1986).

24   Schirrmacher, V.; Ahlert, T.; Heicappell, R. et al.: Successful application of non-oncogenic viruses for antimetastatic cancer immunotherapy. Cancer Rev. *5:* 19–49 (1986).

25   Storch, E.; Kirchner, H.; Schirrmacher, V.: Prolonged survival of mice against the Eb and ESb lymphoma by treatment with interferon inducers alone or in combination with corynebacterium parvum. Cancer Immunol. Immunother. *23:* 179–184 (1986).

26   Vlodavsky, I.; Schirrmacher, V.; Ariav, Y.; Fuks, Z.: Lymphoma cell interaction with cultured vascular endothelial cells and with the subendothelial basal lamina: Attachment, invasion and morphological appearance. Invasion Metastasis *3:* 81–97 (1983).

27   Vlodavsky, I.; Fuks, Z.; Bar-Ner, M. et al.: Lymphoma cell-mediated degradation of sulfated proteoglycans in the subendothelial extracellular matrix: Relationship to tumor cell metastasis. Cancer Res. *43:* 2704–2711 (1983).

28   Hoegen, P. von; Weber, E.; Schirrmacher, V.: Viral xenogenization increases the frequency of cytotoxic T lymphocytes specific for a tumor associated transplantation antigen (submitted for publication).

Prof. Dr. V. Schirrmacher, Institut für Immunologie und Genetik, Deutsches Krebsforschungszentrum, Im Neuenheimer Feld 280, D-6900 Heidelberg (FRG)

Contr. Oncol., vol. 30, pp. 28–41 (Karger, Basel 1988)

Diagnostic Imaging of Lung Metastases

S. J. Tuengerthal

Hospital for Thoracic Diseases, Heidelberg, FRG

The interest in recognition of lung metastases is increasing. In the past, involvement of both lungs with metastatic disease was felt to exclude curative treatment. During the last decade new regimens of cancer therapy have been developed which show promising results. Even multiple lung metastases originating from different tumors have been successfully treated with a 5-year survival time [3, 4, 11, 12, 23, 24]. However, treatment planning requires the early detection of all, even small, lung metastases. Despite the advances of modern chemotherapy, surgery offers the best chance for successful treatment [25–27]. Thus careful monitoring of the patient is indispensible. The failure to detect a pulmonary metastasis can delay the early initiation of a therapeutic regimen and may be fatal. The patient's survival depends on the ability of the physician to detect the metastatic lesion of the lung. The imaging procedures established for diagnosis and follow-up of patients suffering from pulmonary involvement of malignant disease are listed in table I.

Conventional Radiology

Radiological examinations remain the basic diagnostic procedures for the detection of lung metastases. The difference in density between lung tissue containing air and the tumor masses causes a difference of absorption of the X-ray beam and results in abnormal pathological patterns.

The first diagnostic step in imaging lung metastasis will generally be the plain chest film [13]. The roentgenologic features listed in table II may be present alone or in a mixed pattern.

Table I. Imaging procedures for lung metastases

X-ray examinations

Conventional X-ray examinations
Plain chest film
Fluoroscopy (spot film)
Tomography
Contrast studies
  Barium swallow
  Bronchography
  Mediastinal phlebography
  Pulmonary arteriography

Digitized radiography
Digital radiography
Computed tomography

Nuclear medicine
Perfusion scan
Ventilation scan
Tumor imaging
  ^{67}-Ga uptake
  ^{131}-J labeled monoclonal antibodies
Positron emission tomography (SPECT)

Magnetic resonance imaging (MRI)

Ultrasound

Chest films are easily standardized, repeated, and evaluated by experienced readers. The procedure is inexpensive and noninvasive, and the radiation dose is low. Chest films are thought to be very sensitive for showing metastases in the normal lung. The spatial resolution is high and singular nodules of 5 mm may be documented. At present 20–30% of positive chest X-rays are diagnosed as being negative, and 2–5% of negative films are called pathologic. In addition, well-trained, experienced readers disagree on the interpretations of the same film 10–20% of time, and intra-observer variations of 5–10% are common. Despite the technological advances that have occurred, these rates of error do not appear to have changed significantly during the last two decades [1].

The main disadvantage of conventional radiography is the limited depth resolution of the film-screen systems. Even large masses may not

Table II. Pathological/radiological pattern of lung metastases (from [14])

	Primary tumor
Miliary	thyroid
	lung
	bone
	sarcomas
	breast
Lymphangitic	stomach
	breast
	pancreas
	lung
	lymphomas and leukemias
	prostate
'golf ball' (25%)	sarcoma
	clear cell carcinoma
	seminoma
Coarse nodular (25%)	oropharynx
	stomach
	thyroid
	female genital tract
	lymphosarcoma
	chorion epithelioma
Subpleural (25%)	breast
	methothelioma (serous or bloody fluid)
Miscellaneous (5%)	esophagus
Pneumonic and peribronchial nodular	breast

be diagnosed, if they are hidden by mediastinal structures. The development of high lattitude films improves recognition of mass lesions on chest radiographs in paramediastinal, retrocardiac and retrodiaphragmatic areas. Nonetheless some disadvantages remain with the conventional radiogram: mass lesions cannot be detected in the airless lung, and metastatic lesions may not be shown if other lung disease is present. Atelectasis, pneumonitis or fibrosis may obscure mass lesions to a certain extent. In these cases sometimes anterior-posterior, oblique or lateral conventional tomography may be useful in differentiating mass lesions from superimposed pathological structures. Shape, size and localization of lung metastases depends on primary tumor histology and on host condition — both influence radiomorphology (table II). Sensitivity and specificity in detecting lung metastases vary, therefore, for different tumors [1, 9].

X-Ray Morphology of Lung Metastases

Multiple coin-like mass lesions ('golf ball type') (fig. 1), without evidence of calcification and a coarse nodular pattern (fig. 2), with or without pleural effusion, are always suspicious signs of the presence of metastatic lung disease. These patterns were found in approximately 75% of all metastatic lesions, showing a preference for different primary tumors (table II) [15]. Irregular or nodular-reticular patterns are characteristic of lymphatic spread of malignant disease, but there is no pathognomonic sign to distinguish these patterns from non-malignant diseases such as pulmonary fibrosis (fig. 3).

The single coin lesion also causes great problems in differential diagnoses. Calcification is thought to be a sign of non-malignancy, but the metastases of colonic carcinoma or osteosarcoma may be associated with calcified nodules or pleura. There is no chance of distinguishing

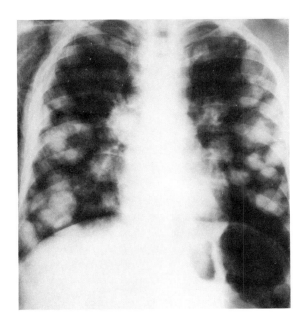

Fig. 1. Golfball-like metastatic lesions; male 48 years. Diagnosis: multiple metastases of malignant seminoma.

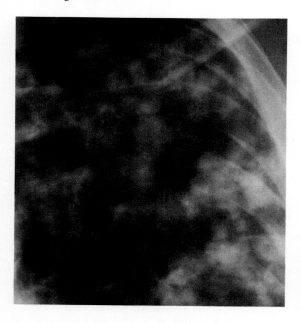

Fig. 2. Coarse nodular-reticular pattern; female 62 years. Diagnosis: metastases of unknown primary tumor (adeno cell carcinoma).

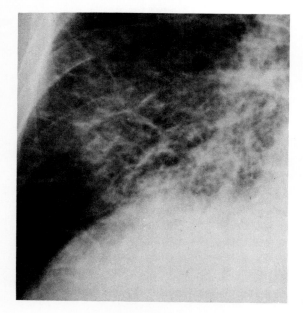

Fig. 3. Reticular pattern which mimics lung tissue fibrosis; male 57 years. Diagnosis: metastases of stomach cancer.

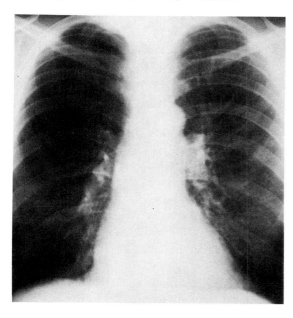

Fig. 4. Unilateral hyperlucent right lung, caused by central airway obstruction due to solitary lung metastasis in the right hilum; female 72 years. Diagnosis: metastatic melanoma.

malignant from non-malignant mass lesions by radiomorphology. Pre-existing chest films can be helpful in distinguishing benign or malignant disease, since lack of growth is thought to signify benign disease in untreated patients.

Lung metastases with a central localization may complicate X-ray findings. In rare instances metastases obliterate bronchi or lung vessels. The following additional X-ray symptoms may occur:

Decreased lung density: due to air being trapped in subtotal bronchial stenosis, overextension of adjacent lung tissue in uncomplicated atelectasis in bronchial occlusion, reduced vessel diameter caused by reflectory mechanism or vascular occlusion (fig. 4).

Increased lung density: due to collapsed lung tissue, lobar or segmental infiltration in the case of obstructive pneumonitis or pulmonary infarction.

Sometimes these X-ray signs are the only manifestation of metastatic involvement of the lung, but these features are non-specific and indistinguishable from other lung disease. They increase the difficulty of arriving at a correct diagnosis. The radiologist has to remember these signs, since they may be the only radiological evidence of malignancy.

Fluoroscopy

Careful fluoroscopic examination of patients with suspected lung metastases remains a worthwhile procedure. The hazard from increased radiation is negligible. Despite a lower spatial resolution compared to film-screen documentation, the fluoroscopic study adds important information. Turning the patient to obtain three-dimensional views during breathing, and observing the organ motion during the Valsalva maneuver increases the sensitivity and specificity in discriminating lung lesions. Pleural or thoracic wall involvement may be documented on spot film under fluoroscopic control. Every radiologist has had the experience of detecting metastases not documented by other imaging methods.

Conventional Linear Tomography

Linear whole-lung tomography may add important information to the plain chest film examination, because it shows more accurately pulmonary involvement of malignant disease [16, 29]. However, diagnostic accuracy is thought to be insufficient, especially in lung areas covered by mediastinal organs. But in comparison to CT the spatial resolution of conventional tomography is higher and small metastases of 3 – 5 mm diameter may be shown, which are not resolvable by CT examination with normal technical configuration. The main disadvantage of tomography is the reduced depth resolution, which obscures paramediastinal, retrocardiac, and retrodiaphragmatic mass lesions. With sufficient compensation filters this handicap can be eliminated, but nevertheless CT will be superior in showing pleural mass lesions (fig. 5).

Contrast Media Investigations

The *barium swallow* under fluoroscopic control should be obtained routinely to document mediastinal tumor spread and assess the esophagus and adjacent mediastinal structures.

Bronchography will only be required rarely after other investigations, including bronchoscopy, conventional tomography and CT, fail to locate a suspected lesion. It then may add important information. The

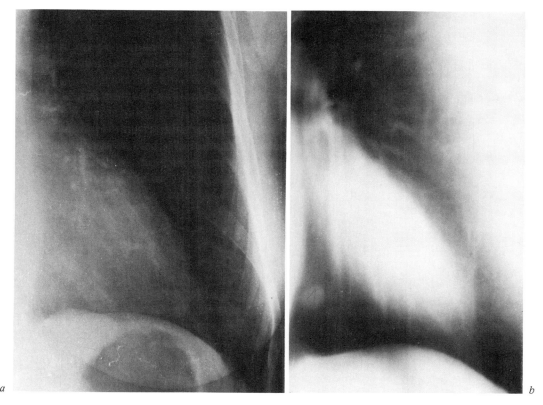

Fig. 5. Small mass lesion in the left lung, not visible on conventional plain chest film, but detected on conventional linear tomography. *a* plain chest film (detail); *b* linear whole lung tomography with anatomically shaped lead-loaded acrylic glass compensation filters (100 my Pb equivalent) (detail). Diagnosis: single lung metastasis of malignant teratoma.

indication may be derived from postoperative chest film or when bleeding occurs due to metastases.

Mediastinal phlebography documents vessel obstruction due to tumor growth within the mediastinum and adds to the information on tumor stage.

The indication for *pulmonary arteriography* in metastatic lung disease is restricted to preoperative staging or for postoperative complications. Several surgeons have demanded arteriographic investigations preoperatively when hilar masses are present or when bronchial and vascular sleeve resections are planned [27].

Bronchial arteriography may be performed in patients with lung metastases when intraarterial chemotherapy or embolization therapy is planned. Most of these invasive contrast investigations are being replaced by other imaging modalities, especially CT.

Digitized Radiography

Digital radiography was introduced in thoracic diagnosis and was assessed for its sensitivity in demonstrating mass lesions. Four technical solutions are now being tested clinically [9, 10]:

  (a) digitized fluoroscopy,
  (b) laser scanning of wide dynamic range films,
  (c) laser scanning of electronic plates,
  (d) multiple detector array technique.

All procedures permit increased depth resolution in comparison to conventional radiography. The display consoles enable the radiologist to vary brightness and contrast. The advantage of digitized radiography for detection of mass lesion on the lung is limited. In comparison to conventional chest films, nodular structures may be detected easily. However, the electronic manipulations reduce spatial resolution. Important morphological details, especially at the border of a mass lesion, may be blurred. Furthermore, it has not been possible to standardize the electronic imaging procedures, so that measurements of single metastases become less accurate. Fraser showed that double-energy subtraction using a prototype digitized chest unit with detector array enabled quantification of the calcium content of pulmonary nodules. But this increased specificity for distinguishing benign from malignant mass lesions is of no value in managing the individual patient [5, 7, 21].

During the last decade *computed tomography (CT)* has become a primary diagnostic procedure for staging patients with malignant tumors. Systems developed with a 512×512 matrix, slice thickness below 0.5 cm, and exposure times of less than 4 seconds, have been shown to be superior for demonstrating tumor spread [2]. CT examinations permit intrapulmonary lung metastases to be detected independently of localization. Particularly helpful are CT investigations which evaluate the retrocardiac and paravertebral regions (fig. 6).

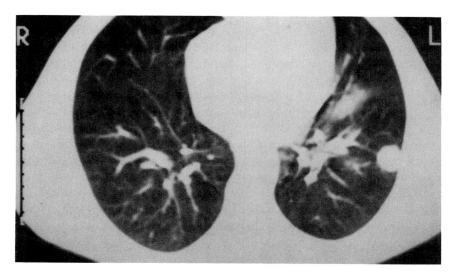

Fig. 6. Single mass lesion on CT examination of the chest (courtesy of Prof. van Kaik, Deutsches Krebsforschungszentrum Heidelberg); male 46 years. Diagnosis: metastasis of left kidney hypernephroma.

Due to increased depth resolution, CT proved advantageous for the detection of thoracic wall involvement, pleural mass lesions, and tumor spread into the mediastinum. In comparison with conventional radiographic chest examinations, CT also shows disadvantages. Conclusive CT investigations are difficult to obtain in non-cooperative patients. Even large basal lung lesions may be missed due to breathing. The spatial resolution is lower than that of the plain film radiographs, and single lung lesions with diameters of less than 8 mm are not visible with most machines used today. Some increase of spatial resolution is possible with a larger matrix size, and with slice thicknesses of less than 5 mm. The radiation dose, however, is increased with these technical modifications. Partial volume effects and motion blurring cause problems with perivascular metastases or lymph node enlargement in the hilar region. CT was shown to be less sensitive than conventional tomography with compensation filters in these areas [17]. Nevertheless, CT examinations are considered superior for diagnostic accuracy [14, 18–20, 22, 29]. The images are easily read, and the documentation of mass lesions, their size and localization, are shown more clearly than on conventional chest film or tomograms. Therefore, clinicians request CT investigations of the thorax for primary tumor staging.

While CT is widely accepted for the initial staging, the procedure is controversial where post-therapy is concerned. CAT scanning is expensive and time-consuming and results in high radiation exposure. In comparison with plain chest films, CT is not cost-efficient [15]. CT should only be performed when clinical data suggest tumor spread [29]. When surgical resection of lung metastases is planned, the surgeon should insist on preoperative CT scanning [27].

Nuclear medicine is not very sensitive in the detection of small mass lesions. Neither ventilation nor perfusion scans are able to detect small lesions (fig. 7 a, b). Both procedures can quantitate obstruction of vessels or bronchi, or may show large lesions. Gallium 67 or thallium 97 scans are only effective with large tumor volume. These isotope procedures will only show lesions which are easily seen with other diagnostic procedures, but they may be helpful in distinguishing coarse interstitial patterns in lymphatic tumor spread. Direct tumor imaging with

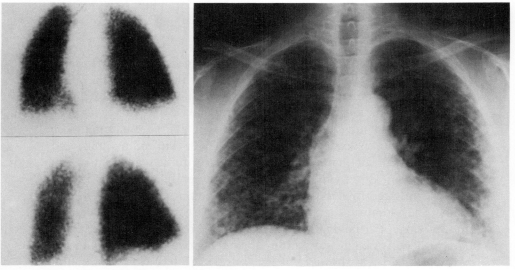

a *b*

Fig. 7. a Perfusion scan posterior-anterior and RAO 45° (courtesy of Prof. van Kaik, Deutsches Krebsforschungszentrum Heidelberg); *b* posterior-anterior plain chest film examination; female 37 years. Diagnosis: multiple lung metastases from undifferentiated ovary carcinoma.

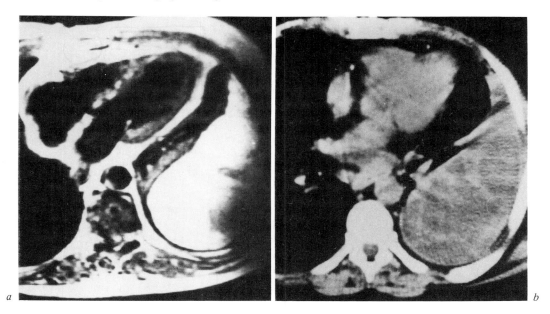

a   *b*

Fig. 8. a MR image; *b* CT examination of the chest; male 56 years. Diagnosis: large intrathoracic metastases (adenocell carcinoma).

monoclonal antibodies and positron emission tomography of the lung (SPECT technique) is today in an experimental stage and as yet without clinical importance [8].

Today *magnetic resonance imaging (MRI)* cannot be recommended for the staging or follow-up of patients with metastatic lung disease. Compared to other imaging modalities, MRI is very expensive. The additional diagnostic information is limited. The exposure time of several minutes induces motion artifacts which diminish the diagnostic information in diaphragmatic and perivascular spaces. The spatial resolution is low. As a result, the information obtained with MRI is lower than with CT investigations (fig. 8 a, b) [39].

Ultrasound is of limited value for detection of pulmonary metastasis, since lung tissue containing air destroys diagnostic information. Only in rare cases will pulmonary lesions situated on the periphery be shown with ultrasound. But it is superior to all other procedures for detecting even small amounts of pleural fluid. Furthermore, ultrasound discriminates radiologically dense areas and permits the differentiation between fluid, atelectasis or tumor spread [6].

Conclusion

For the detection of lung metastases a plain chest film combined with other conventional X-ray procedures such as fluoroscopy and linear tomography is the basic diagnostic imaging procedure. Plain chest films should be obtained according to ILO regulations, but with high latitude films. During primary staging, negative chest films require an additional CT examination. CT is not cost-efficient for post-therapy examinations and should only be requested on clinically selected cases. However, it appears to be necessary prior to metastatic surgery, to document lesions more clearly. All other newly developed imaging procedures − magnetic resonance, sonography, scintigraphy and tumor imaging with labeled monoclonal antibodies − are of minor importance in detecting the early spread of metastases.

References

1   Brogdon, B. G.; Kelsey, C. A.; Moseley, R. D.: Factors affecting perception of pulmonary lesions. Radiol. Clin. N. Am. 21: 633−654 (1983).

2   Chang, A. E.; Schaner, E. G.; Conkle, D. M.: Evaluation of computed tomography in the detection of pulmonary metastasis. Cancer 43: 913−916 (1979).

3   Cliffton, E. E.; Pool, J. L.: Treatment of lung metastases in children with combined therapy. J. thorac. cardiovasc. Surg. 54: 403−412 (1967).

4   Chosksi, L. B.; Takita, H.; Vincent, R. G.: The surgical management of solitary pulmonary metastasis. Surgery Gynec. Obstet. 134, 479−482 (1972).

5   Fraser, E. G.; Breatnach, E.; Bearnes, G. T.: Digital radiography of the chest: clinical experience with a prototyp unit. Radiology 148: 1−5 (1983).

6   Goddard, P.: Indications for ultrasound of the chest. J. thorac. Imag. 1: 89−97 (1985).

7   Godwin, J. D.; Speckman, J. M.; Fram, E. K. et al.: Distinguishing benign from malignant pulmonary nodules by computed tomography. Radiology 144: 349−351 (1982).

8   Hughes, J. M. B.; Brundin, L. H.; Valind, S. O.; Rhodes, C. G.: Positron emission tomography in the lung. J. thorac. Imag. 1: 77−88 (1985).

9   Johnson, G. A.; Ravin, C. E.: A survey of digital chest radiography. Radiol. Clin. N. Am. 21: 655−664 (1983).

10 Merritt, Ch. R. B.; Metthews, Ch. C.; Scheinhorn, D.; Balter, S.: Digital imaging of the chest. J. thorac. Imag. 1: 1−13 (1985).

11 Martini, N.; McCormack, P. M.; Shields, Th. Q.: Secondary tumors in the lung; in Shields, General thoracic surgery, pp. 780−789 (Febinger, Philadelphia 1983).

12 McCormack, P. M.; Martini, N.: The changing role of surgery in pulmonary metastases. Ann. thor. Surg. 28: 139−147 (1979).

13   Milne, E. N. C.: The conventional chest radiograph − does it have future? Appl.
      Radiol. *14:* 13−14 (1985).
14   Meschan, I.: Synopsis of analysis of roentgen signs in general radiology, p. 303.
      (Saunders, Philadelphia, London, Toronto 1976).
15   Muhm, J. R.; Brown, L. R.; Cowe, J. K. et al.: Comparison of whole lung tomo-
      graphy and computed tomography for detecting pulmonary nodules. Am. J.
      Roentg. *131:* 981−984 (1978).
16   Muhm, R. J.: Current place of plain-chest-film tomography in chest disease. J.
      thorac. Imag. *1:* 32−38 (1985).
17   Müller, H. A.; Kaick, G. van; Lüllig, H. et al.: Indikationen zur Computertomo-
      graphie der Lunge und des Mediastinums. Prax. Pneumol. *35:* 213−219 (1981).
18   Osborne, D. R.; Korobkin, M.; Ravin, C. E. et al.: Comparison of plain radio-
      graphy, conventional tomography and computed tomography in detecting intra-
      thoracic lymph node metastasis from lung carcinoma. Radiology *142:* 157−161
      (1982).
19   Schaner, E. G.; Chang, A. E.; Doppmann, L. J. et al.: Comparison of computed
      tomography and conventional whole lung tomography in detecting pulmonary
      nodules: a prospective radiologic pathologic study. Am. J. Roentg. *131:* 51−54
      (1978).
20   Siegelman, S. S.; Zerhouni, E. A.; Leo, F. P. et al.: CT of the solitary pulmonary
      nodule. Am. J. Roentg. *135:* 1−13 (1980).
21   Sommer, F. G.; Smathers, R. L.; Wheat, R. L. et al.: Digital processing of film
      radiographs. Am. J. Roentg. *144:* 191−196 (1985).
22   Sonoda, M.; Takano, M.; Miyahara, J. et al.: Computed radiography utilizing
      scanning laser stimulated luminescence. Radiology *148:* 833−838 (1983).
23   Takita, H. F.; Edgerton, F.; Merrin, C. et al.: Management of multiple lung metas-
      tasis. J. surg. Oncol. *12:* 199−205 (1979).
24   Thomford, N. R.; Woolner, L. B.; Clagett, O. T.: The surgical treatment of metas-
      tasis in the lungs. Surgery, St. Louis *49:* 357−363 (1965).
25   Turney, S. Z.; Haight, C.: Pulmonary resection for metastatic neoplasms. Surgery,
      St. Louis *61:* 784−791 (1971).
26   Vogt-Moykopf, I.; Meyer, F.; Merkle, N. M. et al.: Late results of surgical treatment
      of pulmonary metastasis. Thorac. cardiovasc. Surgeon *34:* 143−148 (1986).
27   Vogt-Moykopf, I.; Meyer, G.: Surgical technique in operations on pulmonary
      metastasis. Thorac. cardiovasc. Surgeon *34:* 125−132 (1986).
28   Wandkte, J. C.; Plewes, D. B.: Chest equilization radiography. J. thorac. Imag. *1:*
      14−20 (1985).
29   Webb, W. R.: Plain radiography and computed tomography in the staging of
      bronchogenic carcinoma: a practical approach. J. thorac. Imag. *2:* 57−65 (1987).
30   Webb, W. R.: Magnetic resonance imaging of the mediastinum, hila and lungs.
      J. thorac. Imag. *1:* 65−73 (1985).

Priv.-Doz. Dr. med. S. J. Tuengerthal, Chefarzt der Röntgenabteilung, Klinik für
Thoraxerkrankungen der LVA Baden, Amalienstraße 5, D-6900 Heidelberg (FRG)

Contr. Oncol., vol. 30, pp. 42–59 (Karger, Basel 1988)

Invasive-Bioptic Diagnosis of Pulmonary Metastases

V. Schulz, G. Meyer, I. Vogt-Moykopf

Hospital for Thoracic Diseases, Heidelberg, FRG

The invasive-bioptic diagnosis of pulmonary metastases is based on various techniques according to the type of manifestation in the lung. The most frequently found coin lesion metastases in the lung periphery, developing from micro-embolisms and, interspersed by the pulmonary arterial system, are mainly dealt with by transthoracic puncture techniques, if not by special bronchoscopic methods or even diagnostic thoracotomy (table I) [14].

This type of peripheral metastases has to be distinguished from central metastases located in the lung core which may appear as lung parenchyma metastases of hematogenous or lymphogenous origin; to some extent endobronchial metastases are involved, originating from spreading tumor cells in the bronchial artery system, or from a lymphangiosis

Table I. Invasive-bioptic methods in the diagnosis of pulmonary metastases; the choice of the method depends on the location of the pulmonary metastases

Location	Invasive-bioptic methods
Central metastases	bronchoscopy (biopsy of endobronchial metastasis; perbronchial puncture of lymphoma by so-called Schießle canula)
	mediastinoscopy
Peripheral metastases	bronchoscopy (aspiration – cytology, Friedel suction biopsy, transbronchial biopsy)
	transthoracic puncture techniques (Hausser, Nordenström)

of the bronchial mucosa, or even from invading lymphoma (fig. 1, 2). As indirect signs of a central metastasis, compressions due to lymphoma extension also have to be taken into consideration. Thus, among the diagnostic procedures to be undertaken in case of central metastases, bronchoscopy should be well to the fore (table I) [14].

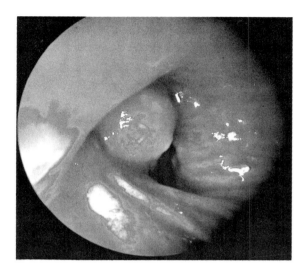

Fig. 1. Endobronchial metastases of a colon carcinoma. The metastases is sitting on the lateral wall of the left main bronchus as a ball-shaped tumor. The medial wall of the left main bronchus is compressed by adjacent lymphoma.

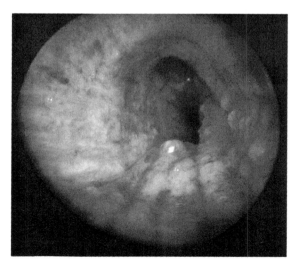

Fig. 2. Small, pinhead-shaped endobronchial metastases of a hypernephroma in the intermediar bronchus.

Bronchoscopy in Central Metastases

Irrespective of the individual visualizing methods for verifying the location of metastases − X-rays, T- and CT scan − endoscopic diagnosis should as a rule start with bronchoscopy. This rule is based on the fact that endobronchial metastases as well as the so-called indirect tumor signs have turned out to be relatively frequent and hence are bound to influence considerably the therapeutic concept − operability, resection procedures − and also the prognosis.

In a group of 295 patients who underwent an operation for pulmonary metastases at our hospital, 15% showed direct or indirect tumor signs in the central bronchial system − up to the segmental bronchus branches (table II). Generally, the reports on the incidence of endobronchial metastases differ extensively. As far as our patients are concerned, an endobronchial metastasis could be established in 4.4%. Baumgartner [1], Hermann [7], and Shepherd [12] report on data showing a rate of between 0 and 40% − also in operated patients. If the number of patients primarily classified as inoperable were to be included, the rate of central bronchial metastases might even be larger.

A scheme depicting the number of endobronchial metastases according to the primary tumor location, based on our own patients as well as on the data of other investigators, shows that the most frequently found metastases are those of mamma carcinomata, followed by those of colorectal carcinomata, and those of kidney and cervix/uterus carci-

Table II. Bronchoscopic findings in the central bronchial system; evaluation of 295 patients with pulmonary metastases (own data)

	n	%
Total of patients	295	100
No verification of metastases	243	82
Indirect signs of metastases	31	11
Direct signs of metastases (endobronchial metastases)	13	4
Not investigated	8	3

Table III. Endobronchial metastases of different primary tumors (own data and data from the literature)

Primary tumor	Own data	Literature data	Total
Mamma	1	44	45
Colorectal	4	20	24
Kidney	2	21	23
Cervix/uterus	—	14	14
Melanoma	—	8	8
Testicle	1	3	4
Thyroid gland	—	3	3
Urinary bladder	—	3	3
Ovary	—	2	2
Suprarenal gland	—	2	2
Fibrosarcoma	—	2	2
Osteosarcoma	1	1	2
Leiomyosarcoma	—	2	2
Bronchus	2	—	2
Pancreas	—	1	1
Prostata	—	1	1
Anal	—	1	1
Penis	—	1	1
Larynx	—	1	1
Synoviasarcoma	1	—	1
Rhabdomysarcoma	1	—	1
Angiosarcoma	—	1	1
Chorion sarcoma	—	1	1
Total	13	132	145

nomata (table III). These absolute data must be accompanied by information on the relative frequency, in order to evaluate the incidence of endobronchial metastases due to a known primary tumor. This procedure proves there is indeed a correlation between absolute and relative data concerning metastases of colorectal and kidney carcinomata, but none in the case of mamma carcinomata. Rare tumors — such as osteosarcomata and testicle teratomata — may on the other hand show a high incidence of endobronchial metastases (table IV).

Bronchoscopy performed with the aid of a fibrescope or rigid instruments has various aims as to the diagnosis of central metastases.

Table IV. Endobronchial metastases of different primary tumors; absolute numbers and relative incidence (own data)

Primary tumor	Total of patients (n)	Indirect signs		Direct signs		Tumor signs total	
		n	%	n	%	n	%
Colorectal carcinoma	25	5	10	4	16	9	36
Hypernephroma	32	5	16	2	6	7	22
Osteosarcoma	28	4	14	1	4	5	18
Testicle teratoma	32	3	10	1	3	4	13
Bronchial carcinoma	10	2	20	2	20	4	40
Cervix carcinoma	12	3	25	—	—	3	25
Mamma carcinoma	34	1	3	1	3	2	6
Synovia carcinoma	14	1	7	1	7	2	14

Histological Diagnosis

Generally, the biopsy of endobronchial metastases is the most convenient method of histological diagnosis, whereas transthoracic puncture or even transbronchial biopsy are much more complicated and troublesome. However, in the case of isolated central endobronchial metastases, bronchoscopy is the only method of achieving a histological diagnosis. In this case, but also if a combination of central and peripheral lesions is under discussion, the histological discrimination of a primary bronchial carcinoma with regard to a second tumor is imperative.

Ascertainment of Operability

Considering the therapeutic concept, the bronchoscopic aspect is of great importance. Even if an operative procedure appears to be the management of choice when one is dealing with pulmonary metastases [16], it may happen that nothing but the result of the bronchoscopy on the extent of a tumor leads to the statement of inoperability. The invasion of lymph node metastases into the tracheal wall, for instance, or the overlapping of bronchial metastases which grow continuously over the main carina into the opposite bronchial system will restrict the operative procedure (fig. 3, 4, 5). The extent to which resectability depends on the bronchoscopic view is underlined by some data evaluated for a group of our own patients: In cases where bronchoscopy had been able to exclude central metastases, an operation with a potentially curative prospect could be carried out in 80% of the patients; where broncho-scopy had proved the incidence of metastases, this procedure could be undertaken only in 6 percent of the patients. The most frequent reason for classifying an operation as not curative was a local inoperability, considering the extent of tumor mass which could not be entirely resect-

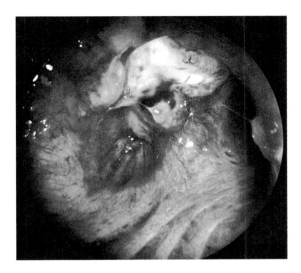

Fig. 3. Lymphoma of a mamma carcinoma penetrate the anterior wall of the trachea near the main carina. The left main bronchus is compressed by lymphoma, partially obturated by invading tumor. The main carina is 'distended'.

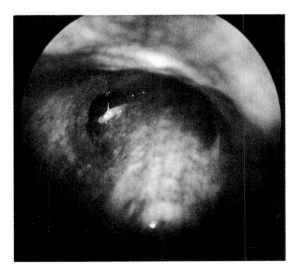

Fig. 4. Pronounced bifurcation syndrome due to hilar and tracheal lymphoma of a mamma carcinoma.

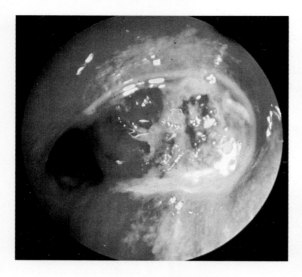

Fig. 5. Metastases of an osteosarcoma in the distal part of the trachea. The metastasis is growing out of the ostium of the right upper lobe and is obturating, peg-shaped, expanding the trachea up to a small lumen on the left side. Since the metastases did not invade the wall of the trachea, the tumor — swinging — obturates the trachea completely when the patient is placed on the left side.

ed. This high percentage of patients who are no longer regarded as radically operable should be an argument — in cases where a central metastasis is supposed — in favor of carrying out an especially critical preoperative staging, even when a local inoperability has been diagnosed.

Resection Procedures

Bronchoscopy on trachea and main bronchi is most decisive if resection procedures concerning pulmonary metastases operations are under consideration. Our results (table V) show that in a group of patients without pathological bronchoscopic findings 71% (n = 179) qualified for parenchyma-conserving surgical interventions as keel and segmental resections, while in cases of central metastases proved by bronchoscopy these procedures were restricted to 34% of the patients (n = 15). Thus 'big operations', including pneumonectomies, bronchoplastic and angioplastic operations, were frequently carried out in this group of patients (table V).

Consideration of Prognosis

In view of the correlations between bronchoscopic diagnosis and operability and resection procedures, it is imaginable that bronchoscopy will also allow a prognosis on disease development: If metastasis removal demands a bronchoplastic or angioplastic extension of the opera-

Table V. Resection procedures based on bronchoscopic findings; evaluation of 295 patients with pulmonary metastases (own data)

Resection procedures	Bronchoscopy: tumor signs (n = 44)		Bronchoscopy: no tumor signs (n = 251)		Factor
	n	%	n	%	
Keel and segmental resection	15	34	179	71	0.5
Enucleation					
Lobectomy	21	47	59	24	2.0
Bilobectomy	6	13.6	4	1.6	8.5
Secondary pneumonectomy	1	2.3	3	1.2	2.0
Pneumonectomy	1	2.3	2	0.8	3.0
Extirpation of mediastinal lymph nodes	—	—	4	2	—
Broncho- and angioplastic operations	16	36	12	4.8	7.5

tion, the prognosis significantly changes for the worse. According to our statistics (fig. 6, 7), the probability of a 3-year survival in this case was only rated at 11%; in a group of patients who underwent standard resections, 51% survived in the same period, a development which is also documented by the two different median survival times of 355 and 1,084 days respectively. If, nevertheless, all visible and palpable tumor masses can be removed, and if bronchoplastic or angioplastic procedures are not required, the survival time is not at all dependent on the registration of central tumor signs. Patients with central metastases documented by bronchoscopy then only have a 'tendency' towards a worse prognosis (fig. 6, 7).

Endoscopic Procedures on Peripheral Pulmonary Metastases

Peripherally located metastases, mostly coin lesions of various shapes, are much more frequently observed than central ones. The relative incidence of peripheral pulmonary metastases due to various pri-

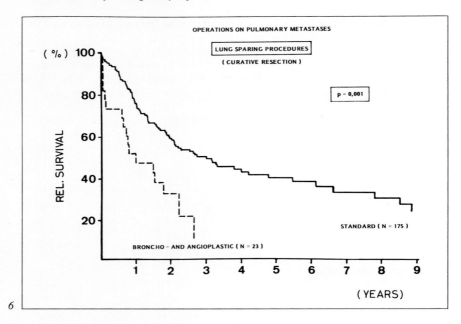

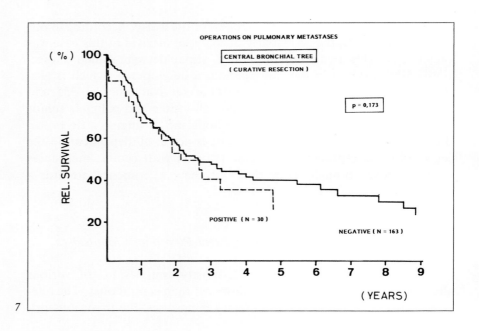

Table VI. Pulmonary metastases of different primary tumors

Localization of primary tumor	Incidence of pulmonary metastases (%)
Hepatoma	20
Esophagus	20– 35
Stomach	20– 30
Pancreas	25– 40
Melanoma	60– 80
Mamma	60
Thyroid gland	65
Hodgkin's syndrome	50– 70
Non-Hodgkin's syndrome	30– 40
Squamous cell carcinoma of neck and head	13– 40
Colon/rectum	20– 43
Ovary	10
Uterus	30– 42
Cervix	20– 30
Vulva	20
Chorion carcinoma	70–100
Kidney	50– 75
Urinary bladder	25– 30
Prostata	13– 20
Testis	70– 80
Penis	10
Wilms' tumor	60
Ewing's sarcoma	77
Neuroblastoma	25
Rhabdomyosarcoma	55
Osteosarcoma	75

Fig. 6. Relative survival rates according to resection procedures (standard resection versus bronchoplastic and angioplastic procedures). Resection procedures were carried out with a potentially curative aim; 198 patients with pulmonary metastases.

Fig. 7. Relative survival rates according to bronchoscopic findings in the central bronchial system. Only standard resections were carried out with a potentially curative aim; 193 patients with pulmonary metastases.

mary tumors can be evaluated by autopsy data (table VI) [19]: Commonly, carcinosarcomata and sarcomata metastasize more frequently into the lung than carcinomata; the first position in the frequency scale is occupied by melanomata, followed by chorion epitheliomata, testicular carcinomata, hypernephromata, Ewing's sarcomata and osteosarcomata, whereas most of the urogenital carcinomata – prostate, penis, vulva and ovarian carcinomata – have only a low tendency to metastasize into the lung.

Any tumor, in theory, is able to metastasize into the lung, even if, as a rule, certain types of tumor show merely a local growth, and metastases are not known. This fact is underlined by the case of a meningioma with pulmonary metastases (fig. 8–9).

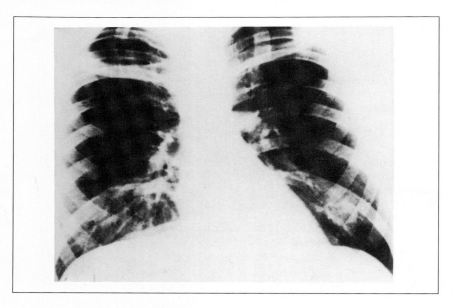

Fig. 8. Chest X-ray. Clearly demarcated circular nodule in the left lower lobe, metastases of a meningioma.

Fig. 9. a Nodular macroscopically well-defined tumor (3×2.8×2.5 cm) in the inferior lobe of the left lung. Identical histological appearance (endotheliomatous meningioma) of *b* lung tumor (needle biopsy; Hausser needle), *c* previously (1976) operated intracranial meningioma, and *d* one of the recently (1981) operated recurrent intracranial meningioma (magnified 500 times).

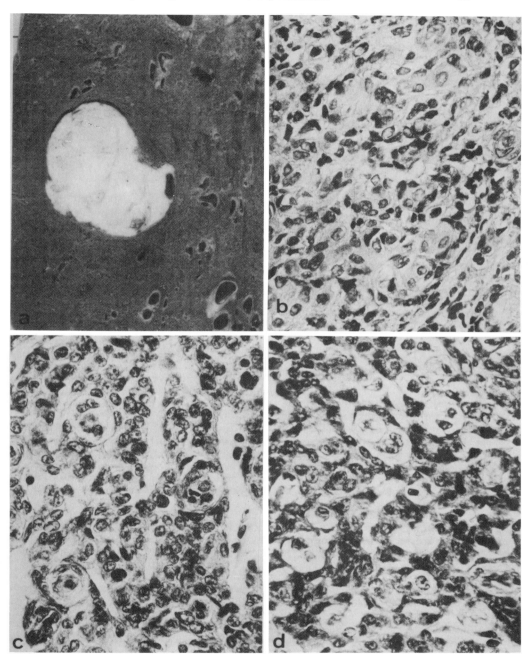

A 38-year-old man was admitted to our ward because of generalized convulsive attacks in intervals of several days. An operation on an olfactory meningioma carried out 5 years earlier suggested that a local relapse of this tumor was the cause of the attacks, which would be proved by CT scan. During pre-operative staging a space in the left lower lobe area was found to be occupied by a lesion, $3 \times 2.8 \times 2.5$ cm in size and with irregular contours. The diagnosis of a second tumor, a peripheral bronchial carcinoma, was obvious. Transthoracic puncture was carried out: the histological data of the biopsy proved a pulmonary metastasis of the known meningioma, which was also confirmed by a specimen taken during operation. A pulmonary metastasis of a meningioma must be regarded as a rarity: up to now only 47 cases have been described in the literature. The relative incidence amounts to approximately $< 0.1\%_0$ (fig. 8−9).

The investigation of peripheral pulmonary metastases may either be performed by bronchoscopic methods, using special techniques of aspiration or biopsy, or by so-called transthoracic puncture techniques. Generally, it is advisable to take the passage through the bronchial system to access the lesions, because the complication rate of this procedure is much lower than that of transthoracic methods. Nevertheless, certain locations such as a focus invading the pleura and infiltrating the thorax wall require transthoracic techniques in any case.

Bronchoscopic Techniques

As for bronchoscopic procedures (table I), aspiration cytology, the so-called Friedel suction biopsy [4], and the transbronchial biopsy can be carried out [3, 18]. The efficiency of aspiration cytology depends on the tumor shape: lesions of a diameter of more than 6 cm can be documented with a relatively high frequency, while smaller ones with a dia-

Table VII. Sensitivity of aspiration cytology in the diagnosis of peripheral pulmonary metastases; the sensitivity depends on the shape of the metastases ('cytological statement' [3])

Diameter	Sensitivity
10−6 cm	35−45%
6−2 cm	15−30%
< 2 cm	< 10%

meter of less than 2 cm show very little diagnostic evidence (table VII) [3]. The histologically verified results concerning the Friedel suction biopsy vary, according to different investigators, within a scale of 15−49%.

In the last few years, transbronchial biopsy has been more and more preferred for diagnosing pulmonary metastases [5]. During X-ray screening and with fibrescopic guidance, a forceps is passed to the peripheral focus, where it takes a biopsy. The success of this procedure depends on whether the lung parenchymal metastasis has grown into the lumen of the small bronchi, or compresses it so that it is accessible to the 'punching' forceps. Data on the efficiency of this procedure, therefore, vary considerably: Wenner et al. [20] report on relevant histological results in 29% of the patients investigated; Ulrichs et al. [15] could diagnose a lung metastasis only in 6% of their patients. When diagnosing a lymphangiosis carcinomatosa, the procedure is at any rate superior to all others; as far as our own experience is concerned, 80−100% of the cases can be diagnosed in this way.

Transthoracic Techniques

Regardless of the puncture instruments applied, transthoracic procedures lead to a high rate of relevant diagnostic results (table VIII). Nevertheless, it must be noted that the punctures documented by our data were performed by well-trained investigators [8, 11, 17, 21].

Table VIII. Results of transthoracic puncture techniques in the diagnosis of peripheral pulmonary metastases.

Author		Method	Patients (n)	Positive results (%)
Vollhaber, 1972	[17]	Hausser	250	91
Zavala and Bedell, 1972	[21]	Travenol	48	80
Paulin et al., 1978	[11]	Aspiration needle	547	75
Paulin et al., 1978	[11]	Hausser	312	87
Jerer and Us-Krasovec, 1980	[8]	Aspiration needle	182	93

The needle mostly employed in Germany was developed by Hausser [6]. By means of this so-called Hausser needle, and following the Menghini principle, tissue cylinders with a diameter of 1 mm and a length of 10 mm can be obtained. Because of their relatively large size, punctures should be restricted to lesions in the lung periphery; this way, hemorrhages of larger pulmonary arteries will be avoided. Such reservations are not required for the Nordenström [9] needle, which is used just as often. The nearly non-traumatic application allows for a smear cytology to be set up and makes it possible to obtain sufficient material for histological investigations. With this needle, it must also be noted in general that clotting disorders, a pulmonary hypertension as well as respiratory insufficiency and state after pneumonectomy contraindicate the application.

The risk of dropping tumor cells along the insertion canal is overestimated. In a group of 1,260 patients, Sinner et al. [13] could only report one single case of cutaneous metastasis caused by such an incident. The data of Nordenström [10] are similar: one patient out of 4,000 developed a tumorous cutaneous infiltration in the puncture area.

Sensitivity of Procedures

Although at first sight the findings obtained by bronchologic techniques – and even more the results of transthoracic procedures – seem to be quite sufficient, a considerable rate of false-negative data must be taken into consideration (table VIII). Even transthoracic punctures lead to false-negative results within a range of 5–15% (table VIII).

This has various reasons: it may happen that during puncture the lesion is missed due to an inadequate radiological view and/or its small size. It may also happen that a metastasis has developed a 'hard peel' so that the needle 'pushes' the tumor ahead. But even if the focus is accessed by puncture, false-negative results are possible: if a necrotic specimen is taken from a rather central site, it will be difficult to obtain a reliable histological result. Another risk of mis-interpretation may exist if inflammatory interstitial lung tissue situated in the periphery of the metastasis has been taken by puncture.

With regard to the false-negative results in question, and considering the various possible complications such as pneumothorax, hemoptysis, and air embolism, all the described invasive methods of diagnosing peripheral pulmonary metastases are of limited sensitivity. Thus, if pulmonary lesions can be verified with sufficient probability as metastases of a known primary tumor still present or previously existing, and if operability has been established according to the criteria of metastasis surgery as well as those of tumor biology, nowadays surgical procedures are as a rule carried out even without pre-operative histological investigation of metastasis etiology.

It might be an argument against this management that even in the presence of a known extrathoracic tumor a pulmonary lesion should not be declared a lung metastasis without having been thoroughly investigated. In a study on more than 800 patients with an extrathoracic tumor, Cahan et al. [2] could prove that lesions found in the lung during the diagnostic procedure or in the later progress were verified as metastases only in 196 of the patients, while 500 patients suffered from a primary bronchial carcinoma, and 16 patients even showed a benign tumor. Nevertheless, these data may not strictly be regarded as reliable, and should not result in operative procedures being rejected without preceding histological verification of pulmonary metastases, as any pulmonary lesions supposed to be tumorous should be primarily dealt with by an operation – insofar as operability has been established according to function and staging criteria.

Considering this demand, transthoracic puncture techniques in particular will have to be restricted to a few indications. The application is warranted if the biology of the primary tumor suggests a conserving therapy to start with. Before treatment the pulmonary metastasis is to be verified by puncture and must be distinguished from inflammatory pseudotumors and other tumors which would require a different therapy. Transthoracic puncture may also be carried out in functionally inoperable patients in order to verify a pulmonary metastasis with regard to therapeutic consequences.

Summing up the invasive-bioptic diagnostic procedures in pulmonary metastases, we come to the following conclusions: Bronchoscopy is obligatory; it proves the presence of central metastases and is able to furnish pre-operative information for operability and resection strategy. Moreover, bronchoscopy may access a peripheral pulmonary metastasis by special techniques, such as aspiratory cytology and transbronchial biopsy. Peripheral lesions may also be dealt with by transthoracic bioptic puncture techniques. The histological verification of a peripheral lesion is not obligatory, particularly in view of possible complications, if operability has been established according to the criteria of metastasis surgery and of primary tumor biology.

Should a conserving therapy be chosen, even in functionally inoperable patients, the peripheral lesion nevertheless has to be diagnosed by biopsy beforehand, if the therapeutic consequences are to be considered.

References

1 Baumgartner, W. A.; Mark, J. B.: Metastatic malignancies from distant sites to the tracheobronchial tree. J. thorac. cardiovasc. Surg. *79:* 499 (1980).

2 Cahen, W. G.; Castro, E. B.; Hajdn, S. J.: The significance of a solitary lung shadow in patients with colon carcinoma. Cancer *33:* 414 (1974).

3 Fletcher, E. C.; Levin, D. C.: Flexible fiberoptic bronchoscopy and fluoroscopically guided transbronchial biopsy in the management of solitary pulmonary nodules. West. J. Med. *136:* 477 (1982).

4 Friedel, H.: Die Katheterbiopsie des peripheren Lungenrundherdes. Tuberkulose-bibliothek Nr. 99 (Barth, Leipzig 1961).

5 Haponek, E. F.; Summer, W. R.; Terry, P. B.; Wang, K. P.: Clinical decision making with transbronchial biopsies. Am. Rev. resp. Dis. *125:* 524 (1982).

6 Hausser, R.: Über die diagnostische gezielte Gewebspunktion bei unklaren Lungen-, Pleura- und Mediastinalprozessen. Dt. med. Wschr. *90:* 1809 (1965).

7 Hermann, A.; Schamann, M.; Spiegel, M.: Endobronchiale Metastasen von extra-thorakalen Malignomen. Schweiz. med. Wschr. *112:* 215 (1982).

8 Jerer, M.; Us-Krasovec, M.: Thin needle biopsy of chest lesions, time-saving potential. Chest *78:* 288 (1980).

9 Nordenström, B.: A new instrument for biopsy. Radiology *117:* 474 (1975).

10 Nordenström, B.; Sinner, W. N.: Needle biopsies of pulmonary lesions. Fortschr. Röntgenstr. *129:* 414 (1978).

11 Paulin, A.; Ferluga, D.; Habic-Paulin, A.: Perthorakale Lungenpunktion in der Diagnostik der Lungentumoren. Prax. Pneumolog. *32:* 480 (1978).

12 Shepherd, M. P.: Endobronchial metastatic disease. Thorax *37:* 362 (1982).

13 Sinner, W. N.; Zajicek, J.: Implantation metastasis after percutaneous transthoracic needle aspiration biopsy. Acta radiol. (Diag.) *17:* 473 (1976).

14 Trendelenburg, F. (ed.): Tumoren der Atmungsorgane und des Mediastinums. A. Allgemeiner Teil. Handbuch der inneren Medizin, vol. 4: Erkrankungen der Atmungsorgane; 5th reprint (Springer, Berlin, Heidelberg, New York, Tokyo 1985).

15 Ulrichs, B.; Richard, Y.; Hoad, S.; Mitchell, A.: Diagnosis of bronchial lesions by fiberoptic bronchoscopy. Chest *81:* 262 (1982).

16 Vogt-Moykopf, I.; Meyer, G.; Bülzebruck, H.: Lungenmetastasen – Therapieindi-kation und chirurgische Technik. Münch. med. Wschr. *128:* 295 (1986).

17 Vollhaber, H. H.: Lungenbiopsie. Schweiz. med. Wschr. *102:* 1440 (1972).

18 Wallace, J. M.; Deutsch, A. L.: Flexible fiberoptic bronchoscopy and percutaneous needle lung aspiration for evaluating the solitary pulmonary nodule. Chest *81:* 665 (1982).

19   Weiss, L.; Gilbert, H. A.: Patterns of pulmonary metastasis. Introduction; in Weiss,
     Gilbert, Pulmonary metastasis, pp. 100–103 (The Hague, Boston, London 1978).
20   Wenner, J.; Stuart, R.; Michels, A.: Transbronchial biopsy in the diagnosis of pul-
     monary metastasis. Br. J. Dis. Chest *74:* 81 (1980).
21   Zavala, D. C.; Bedell, G. N.: Percutaneous lung biopsy with a cutting needle. Am.
     Rev. resp. Dis. *106:* 186 (1972).

Prof. Dr. V. Schulz, Internistisch-Pneumologische Abteilung, Krankenhaus
Rohrbach, Klinik für Thoraxerkrankungen der LVA Baden, Amalienstraße 5,
D-6900 Heidelberg (FRG)

Contr. Oncol., vol. 30, pp. 60–75 (Karger, Basel 1988)

Diagnostic Efficiency of Tumor Marker Analyses in Patients with Pulmonary Metastases

W. Ebert, H. O. Werling, H. Bülzebruck, Ö. L. Schönberger

Hospital for Thoracic Diseases, Heidelberg, FRG

Introduction

The measurement of tumor-related substances is playing an increasingly important role in clinical oncology. The most widely used tumor markers are CEA, AFP, HCG, calcitonin, and prostatic acid phosphatase [11].

CEA as an antigen specific for adenocarcinoma of the digestive tract was first demonstrated by Gold and Freedman in 1965. In the following years it became obvious that CEA was produced in a large variety of cancers of epithelial origin including colorectal, pancreatic, gastric, lung, and breast cancer [9].

The tumor marker AFP was found in humans with hepatocellular carcinoma [14] and germ cell neoplasms [1], whereas HCG turned out to be an important factor in the diagnosis of gestational trophoblastic tumors in women [2] and testicular germ cell tumors [12].

We investigated the diagnostic reliability of CEA, AFP, and HCG in the management of patients with pulmonary metastases of different primary tumors.

The purpose of this study was to address the following questions: Do the markers point to the localization and histology of the primary tumor? Are the markers helpful in recording the course of the disease from the viewpoint of treatment response and subsequently of tumor recurrence and progression?

Are pretherapeutic marker determinations of any value in predicting outcome of the disease?

Material and Methods

In 1984/85 381 patients with pulmonary metastases of different primary tumors were admitted for therapy to the Hospital for Thoracic Diseases in Heidelberg/Rohrbach.

CEA was measured in the sera of 238 patients (= 62.7%) by commercially available enzyme immunoassay (CEA Roche, Basel, Switzerland). AFP and β-HCG were tested in the sera of 13 patients with metastasizing testicular teratocarcinomas by commercially available radioimmunoassay (Amersham, Buchler, Braunschweig, FRG).

The classification of the histologic tumor cell type was performed according to the WHO criteria.

Calculation of survival rates was performed using the Kaplan and Meier estimation [10]. The differences in the survival rates were subjected to the log-rank test [13].

Results

The amount of CEA in the sera of 238 patients with pulmonary metastases of different primary tumors prior to therapy was determined. The results are shown in figures 1 and 2. By applying a cut-off

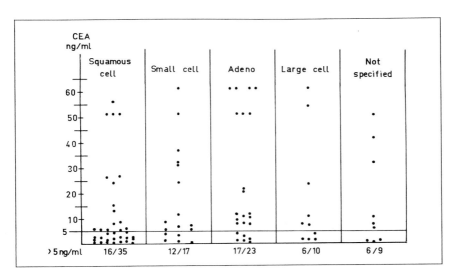

Fig. 1. CEA levels in patients with pulmonary metastases of bronchial carcinoma in relation to histologic cell types.

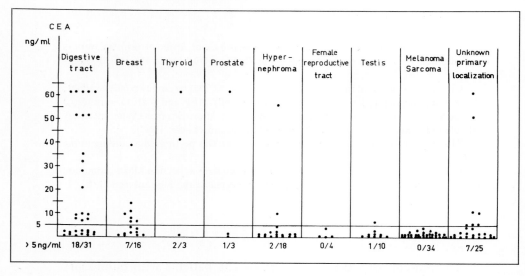

Fig. 2. CEA levels in patients with pulmonary metastases of different primary tumors.

point of 5 ng/ml CEA to discriminate between malignant and benign disease, elevated CEA values were found in 39.9% of all cases.

The sensitivity in detecting malignancy with the CEA assay varied depending on the primary tumor (table I). The CEA assay is most sensitive for carcinoma of the digestive tract followed by bronchial and breast carcinoma.

CEA levels in sarcoma, melanoma, and testicular carcinoma, however, were found to be within the normal range. Furthermore, carcinoma of the kidney showed increased CEA values only in 2 out of 18 cases.

Elevated CEA levels were found in all major histologic tumor cell types of bronchial carcinoma. The highest values of tumor sensitivity were shown by adeno and small cell carcinoma. By applying the Kruskal-Wallis test in combination with multiple comparisons according to Dunn, elevated CEA values showed no statistically significant differences with respect to the cell types.

For comparison, the results of a previous study of CEA analysis in bronchial cancer without pulmonary metastases into the contralateral lung are additionally listed in table I [5]. As can be seen, the sensitivity

Table I. Diagnostic sensitivity of tumor marker assays in patients with pulmonary metastases

	Sensitivity	
	*without**	*with pulmonary metastases*
CEA		
cut-off level: 5 ng/ml		
Bronchial carcinoma (total)	31.6%	60.6%
Squamous cell	29.0%	45.7%
Adeno	54.2%	73.9%
Small cell	38.1%	70.6%
Large cell	55.6%	60.0%
Pulmonary metastases of		
Gastrointestinal carcinoma	58.1%	
Breast carcinoma	43.8%	
Hypernephroma	11.1%	
Testicular teratocarcinoma	10.0%	
Melanoma, Sarcoma	0.0%	
AFP		
cut-off level: 12 ng/ml		
Pulmonary metastases of testicular teratocarcinoma	92.3%	
β-HCG		
cut-off level: 5 mU/ml		
Pulmonary metastases of testicular teratocarcinoma	46.2%	

* Data from a previous study [5]

values of CEA in bronchial carcinoma with pulmonary metastases are higher, thus reflecting the enhancement of malignant disease in metastasizing carcinoma.

Serial CEA determinations were done before and after surgery and during chemotherapy. For metastasizing bronchial carcinoma 19 courses had been registered. In 14 cases (= 73.7%) a decline of CEA values after initial metastasis therapy was observed (fig. 3). Similar results were obtained with other metastasizing primary tumors. After

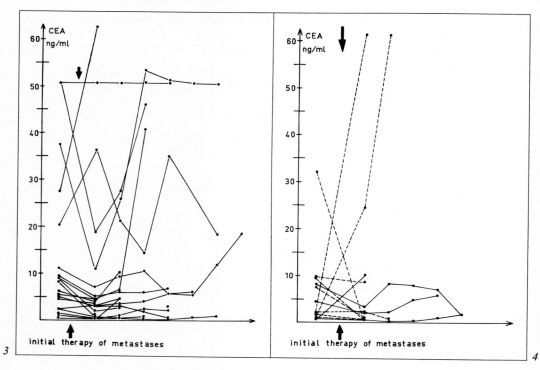

Fig. 3. Serial CEA levels in patients with pulmonary metastases of bronchial carcinoma.

Fig. 4. Serial CEA levels in patients with pulmonary metastases of gastrointestinal and breast carcinoma.

the beginning of therapy the CEA values decreased in 9 out of 12 patients suffering from metastasizing breast and colorectal carcinoma (fig. 4).

It should be stressed that in 3 cases with an increase of CEA the serum sample was obtained up to one year after surgery, so an initial decrease in the CEA level could not be detected. These few cases showed us that it is necessary to measure CEA within a shorter period.

As shown in figure 5, CEA determinations every other month after surgery provide valuable information on the efficacy of the treatment. After resection of an adenocarcinoma of the colon, elevated CEA

($>$ 50 ng/ml, not shown in fig. 5) returned to normal range. After a short period of normal levels a progressive rise of CEA was accompanied by recurrences in lung and liver.

Surgical removal of metastases together with adjuvant chemotherapy led to a decrease of CEA, which reached normal values for some months. But after a period of clinical remission CEA titers increased although the chemotherapy schema was changed. After repeated changes of chemotherapy the patient responded to therapy and CEA decreased.

The other two tumor markers AFP and β-HCG were measured in the sera of 13 patients with pulmonary metastases of testicular teratocarcinoma. Twelve out of 13 patients (= 92.3%) had elevated AFP values, whereas β-HCG was only enhanced in 6 patients (= 46.2%) (table I).

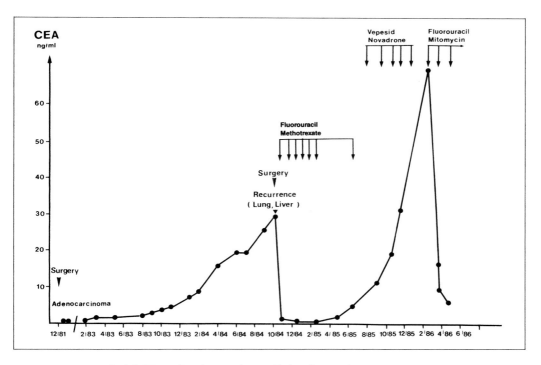

Fig. 5. Serial CEA values in a patient suffering from pulmonary metastases of an adenocarcinoma of the colon during therapy.

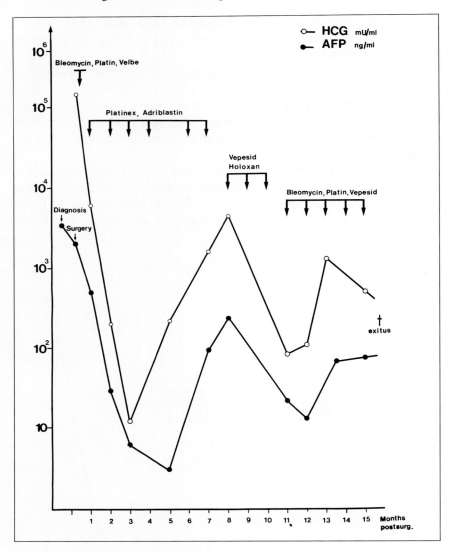

Fig. 6. Serial AFP and β-HCG values in a patient with pulmonary metastases of a testicular teratocarcinoma during chemotherapy.

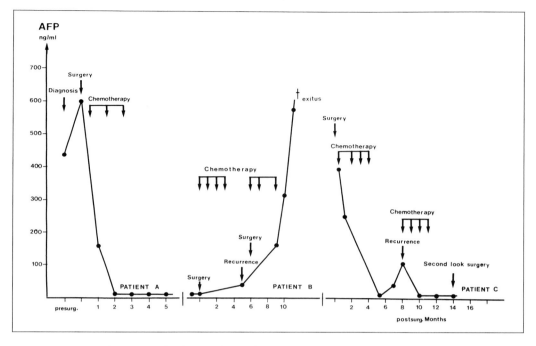

Fig. 7. Serial AFP levels in patients with pulmonary metastases of testicular terato-carcinomas during therapy.

Serial determinations of AFP and β-HCG are potential aids in monitoring the effect of therapy on tumor activity, as can be seen in figures 6 and 7. AFP and β-HCG levels provided a good correlation with both surgical excision and chemotherapy response. The markers also predicted relapse, with increasing markers seen before clinical evidence of recurrence.

To evaluate the significance of CEA as a prognostic factor, the marker was measured in 99 patients with pulmonary metastases before treatment. The survival time of patients was calculated from the beginning of therapy until death or until the last data of observation of the survivors. As expected, the patients suffering from small or large cell carcinoma showed a worse prognosis compared to the other patients (table II, fig. 8).

Table II. Overall survival in relation to histological tumor cell types

| | Histologic cell type | | | | | |
	squamous cell carcinoma	small cell carcinoma	adeno-carcinoma	large cell carcinoma	mixed types	not specified	total
Number of patients							
examined	29	13	38	9	2	8	99
Alive	10	2	18	2	1	3	36
Died	19	11	20	7	1	5	63
% Survival	34.5	15.4	47.4	22.2	50.0	37.5	36.4

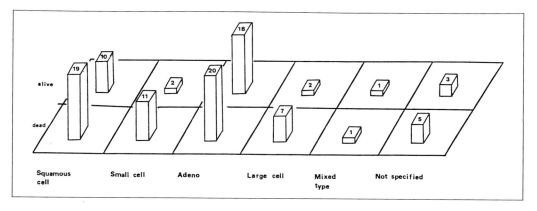

Fig. 8. Overall survival in relation to histological tumor cell type.

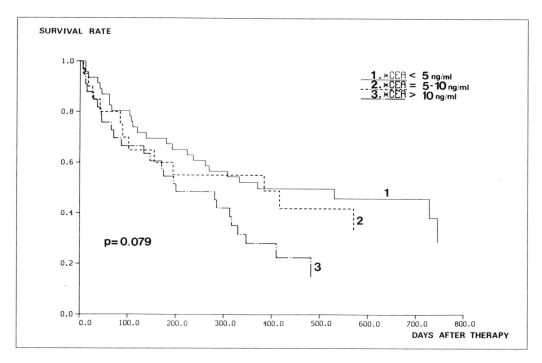

Fig. 9. Survival of patients with pulmonary metastases of bronchial carcinoma of all histologic tumor cell types in relation to CEA levels (0−5, 5−10, > 10 ng/ml) prior to initial metastases therapy.

The survival rate, calculated with the Kaplan and Meier plot with pretherapeutic CEA levels ranging from 0–5, 5–10, > 10 ng/ml, respectively, is shown in figure 9. The differences are not statistically significant (p = 0.079).

However, a significant difference in survival rate (p = 0.026) can be seen between the patients with a pretherapeutic CEA level of less than 10 ng/ml and above 10 ng/ml (fig. 10).

The 66 patients with a CEA level below 10 ng/ml had an increased median survival of 385 days in contrast to 201 days for the 33 patients with CEA levels above 10 ng/ml.

Because prognosis depends largely on the histologic cell type and because these patients had the worst prognosis of small cell or large cell carcinoma, their CEA values have been excluded. Thus, the estimation of survival rate according to the CEA level below and above 10 ng/ml

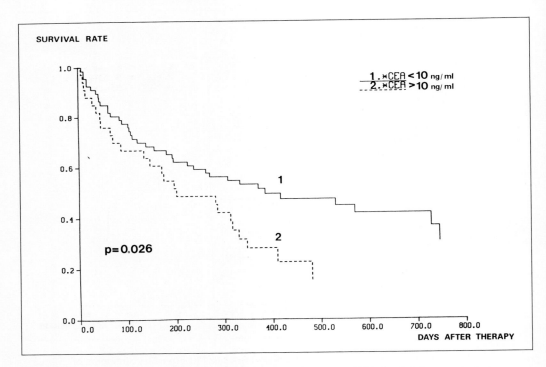

Fig. 10. Survival of all patients according to a CEA level below and above 10 ng/ml.

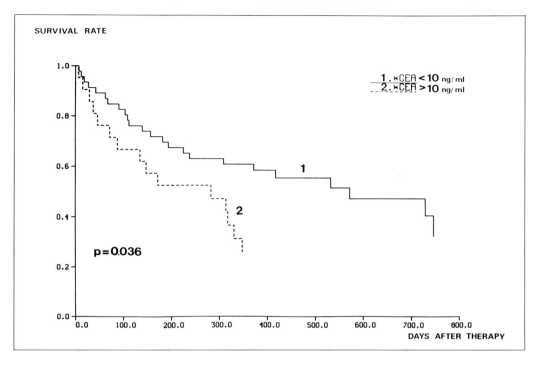

Fig. 11. Survival of the patients suffering from squamous cell carcinoma and adenocarcinoma according to a CEA level below and above 10 ng/ml.

revealed an increased median survival time for the 67 patients suffering from squamous cell and adenocarcinoma. The 46 patients with CEA levels below 10 showed a median survival time of 571 days, whereas the survival rate of the 21 patients above 10 ng/ml increased to 282 days. These differences are statistically significant ($p = 0.036$, fig. 11).

The estimation of survival rate of the 29 patients sufering from squamous cell carcinoma revealed a median survival time of 237 days for those below 10 ng/ml and 87 days for the patients above 10 ng/ml ($p = 0.034$, fig. 12).

Computing the survival rate for 38 patients with adenocarcinoma resulted in the longest median survival time of 746 days for the patients with CEA values below 10 ng/ml and 317 days for those with higher CEA values ($p = 0.039$, fig. 13).

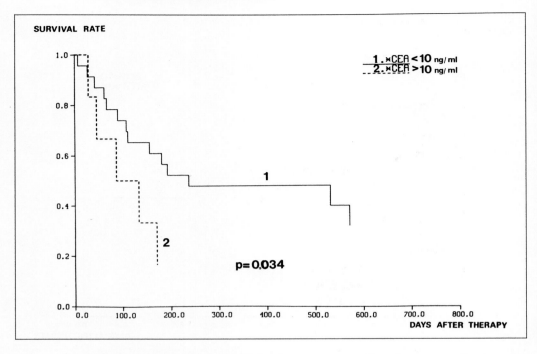

Fig. 12. Survival of patients suffering from squamous cell carcinoma according to a CEA level below and above 10 ng/ml.

Discussion

The results of CEA, AFP, and HCG determinations demonstrate that marker studies are useful parameters for clinical evaluation in the diagnosis and monitoring of patients with pulmonary metastases of primary tumors of different organs. Elevated CEA levels were detected in up to 60.6% of metastasizing bronchial carcinoma, in 58.1% of colorectal carcinomas, and in 43.8% of breast carcinomas. With the exception of very few cases, CEA values in metastasizing melanoma, sarcomas, testicular carcinomas, and carcinoma of the kidney were found to be within the normal range. Thus, it does not appear to be productive to look for CEA as a marker in these malignant diseases [11]. CEA levels were found to be elevated in all cell types of metastasizing bronchial carcinoma but with different magnitudes. However, the differences are not statistically significant, confirming previous findings by Goslin et

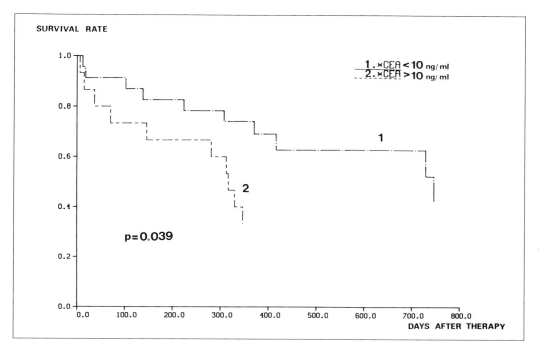

Fig. 13. Survival of patients suffering from adenocarcinoma according to a CEA level below and above 10 ng/ml.

al. [7] and Ebert et al. [5]. The calculated values of sensitivity of CEA in detecting cancer were found to be higher in patients with pulmonary metastases compared to those without metastasizing into the contralateral lung. This is in accordance with data from a previous study of CEA analyses in 500 patients with histologically proved bronchial carcinoma and 500 patients with benign discorders: By applying the Jonckheere test a statistically high significant trend of CEA values depending on TNM staging was found [5].

About 41.8% of patients with primary bronchial, colorectal, and breast carcinomas do not have elevated CEA values. Such false negatives may be related to the degree of tumor differentiation. Poorly differentiated carcinomas tend to be associated with a reduced proclivity to CEA expression and release [4]. Other factors have also been shown to be important in the degree of CEA elevation, including the ability to enter the circulation and the rate of hepatic clearance [15].

The levels for the other two tumor markers were also increased. An elevated amount of AFP was present in up to 94% of metastasizing testicular carcinomas.

Abnormal HCG levels have been shown in up to 46% in those malignancies. Waldman and McIntire [19] have stated that elevation of one or both markers can be expected in 80–90% of patients with nonseminomatous germ cell tumors.

Serial determinations of CEA, AFP, and HCG in patients with marker production were also useful in monitoring response to therapy and in predicting relapse. Increased marker levels declined with response to treatment. A progressive rise during therapy indicated relapse and a need to change therapy. The increasing levels anticipated clinical evidence of recurrence by several months. The observations clearly demonstrate that sequential marker analyses should be performed at very short intervals to obtain optimal surveillance of patients with pulmonary metastases. The interval can be increased when the clinical response is less dramatic and when the markers have returned to within normal range.

Our findings confirm follow-up studies of patients with lung cancer reported by Vincent and Chu [16], Vincent et al. [18], Gropp et al. [8] and Goslin et al. [7].

Pretherapeutic CEA determinations are of some prognostic value. Concannon et al. [3] have shown that preoperative CEA levels are of prognostic value in patients with epidermoid and adenocarcinoma of the lung who have values > 6 ng/ml, since all of these patients have died within less than 3 years and all of the long-term survivors (3–5 years) had levels ≤ 6 ng/ml.

Vincent et al. [17] have stated that a CEA level ≥ 15 ng/ml should raise grave doubts as to the probability of a successful resection in patients with bronchogenic carcinoma for whom a surgical procedure is being considered.

Our study indicates a correlation between pretherapeutic CEA values and outcome of the disease, insofar as patients whose pretherapeutic CEA levels are at the lower end of the spectrum have better survival rates than patients whose levels are in excess of 10 ng/ml.

References

1   Abelev, G. I.: Alpha-fetoprotein in ontogenesis and its association with malignant tumors. Adv. Cancer Res. *14:* 295–358 (1971).

2 Bagshawe, K. D.: Risk and prognostic factors in trophoblastic neoplasia. Cancer *38:* 1373–1385 (1976).

3 Concannon, J. P.; Dalbow, M. W.; Hodsson, S. E.: Prognostic value of preoperative CEA plasma levels in patients with bronchogenic carcinoma. Cancer *42:* 1477–1483 (1978).

4 Denk, H.; Tappeiner, G.; Eckerstorfer, R.: CEA in gastrointestinal and extra-gastrointestinal tumors and its relationship to tumor cell differentiation. Int. J. Cancer *10:* 262–272 (1972).

5 Ebert, W.; Werling, H. O.; Isele, J.; Kayser, K. W: Tumor markers CEA and NSE in lung cancer. Quim. Clin. *5:* 235 (1986).

6 Gold, P.; Freedman, S. O.: Specific carcinoembryonic antigens of the human digestive system. J. exp. Med. *122:* 467–481 (1965),

7 Goslin, R. H.; Skarin, A. T.; Zamcheck, N.: CEA: a useful monitor of therapy of small cell lung cancer. JAMA *246:* 2173–2176 (1981).

8 Gropp, C.; Havemann, K.; Schener, A.: The use of CEA and peptide hormones to stage and monitor patients with lung cancer. J. Radiat. Oncol. Biol. Phys. *6:* 1047–1053 (1980).

9 Hansen, H. J., Snyder, L. J., Miller, E.: CEA assay. A laboratory adjunct in the diagnosis and management of Cancer. J. hum. Pathol. *5:* 139–147 (1974).

10 Kaplan, E. L.; Meier, P.: Nonparametric estimation from incomplete observations. J. Am. stat. Assoc. *53:* 447–454 (1958).

11 McIntire, K. R.: Tumor markers; in DeVita, Hellmann, Rosenberg, Cancer principles and practice of oncology; 2nd edition, pp. 375–388 (Lippincott, Philadelphia 1985).

12 Moore, M. R.; Vogel, C. L.; Watton, K. N.: Use of human chorionic gonadotropin and alpha-fetoprotein in evaluation of testicular tumors. Surg. Gynecol. Obstet. *147:* 167–174 (1978).

13 Peto, R.; Peto, J.: Asymptomatically efficient rank invariant test procedures. J. Roy. Statist. Soc. A *135:* 185–206 (1972).

14 Tatarinov, Y. S.: Presence of embryo-specific alpha-globulin in the serum of patients with primary hepatocellular carcinoma. Vopr. Med. Khim. *10:* 90–91 (1964).

15 Thomas, P.; Hems, D. A.: The hepatic clearance of circulating native and asialo CEA by the rat. Biochem. biophys. Res. Commun. *67:* 1205–1209 (1975).

16 Vincent, R. G.; Chu, T. M.: CEA in patients with carcinoma of the lung. J. Thorac. Cardiovasc. Surg. *66:* 320–328 (1973).

17 Vincent, R. G.; Chu, T. M.; Fergen, T. B.; Ostrander, M.: CEA in 228 patients with carcinoma of the lung. Cancer *36:* 2069–2076 (1975).

18 Vincent, R. G.; Chu, T. M.; Lane, W. W.; Gutierrez, A. C.; Stegemann, R. N.; Madajewicz, S.: CEA as a monitor of successful surgical resection in 130 patients with carcinoma of the lung. J. thorac. cardiovasc. Surg. *75:* 734–739 (1978).

19 Waldmann, R. A.; McIntire, K. R.: The use of sensitive assays for alpha-feto-protein in monitoring the treatment of malignancy; in Heberman, McIntire, Immundiagnosis of cancer (Marcel Dekker, New York, 1979).

Prof. Dr. W. Ebert, Krankenhaus Rohrbach, Thoraxklinik der LVA Baden, Amalienstraße 5, D-6900 Heidelberg 1 (FRG)

Contr. Oncol., vol. 30, pp. 76–107 (Karger, Basel 1988)

Indications and Long-Term Results in Surgery of Pulmonary Metastases

I. Vogt-Moykopf[a], G. Meyer[a], H. Bülzebruck[b], N. M. Merkle[a], M. Langsdorf[a]

[a] Surgical Department and
[b] Department of Medical Documentation, Statistics and Data Processing, Rohrbach Hospital, Hospital for Thoracic Diseases, Heidelberg, FRG

Introduction

Besides the local growth of primary tumor or recurrence, the fate of the oncological patient is determined by the development of distant metastases, which until the recent past was regarded as an unfavorable disease manifestation.

With a more aggressive concept of therapy in the interdisciplinary oncological collaboration of medical oncologists, radiologists and surgeons, a proportion of the patients can today be offered meaningful help, and there is indeed the prospect of cure in a small but increasing percentage.

Besides the nature and number of organs affected by metastases, in the first instance the histological type of the primary tumor, its localization, and its biological behavior are primarily decisive for the prospects of success.

Pulmonary metastases are problems of particular significance in purely quantitative terms. On the basis of information obtained epidemiologically from autopsy statistics, the lung is the most frequent site of metastatic spreading, accounting for about 30% of patients who have died of malignancies [50]. In more than 20% of cases, additional organ metastases other than in the lungs are not found [14]. It is to be assumed that at an earlier stage of the disease an isolated metastatic spreading in the lungs is present in a much higher percentage. This can be dealt with surgically with a view to cure. In particular, kidney, testis, breast, prostate, and cervix carcinomas (i. e., tumors from the genito-urinary tract) show this tendency. For osteosarcomas and soft-tissue sarcomas, it is known that the lungs constitute the sole site of early metastatic spreading in more than 90% of the cases [36].

Although surgical treatment of pulmonary metastases may be regarded as an established technique today, its worldwide spreading has increased rapidly only in the past 10–20 years. The beginnings of surgery of pulmonary metastases extend farther back than those of primary tumor surgery: in 1855 Sedillot performed the first pulmonary resection for a metastasis [25]. Weinlechner [47] and Krönlein [18] reported in 1882 and 1884 on the removal of a pulmonary metastasis discovered by chance during a chest wall resection for a sarcoma. Röpke [35] carried out the first planned lobectomy in 1921 for a metastasis of a breast cancer operated on three years previously. In 1927, Divis [9] described the removal of a solitary pulmonary metastasis of a soft-tissue sarcoma. In 1939, Barney and Churchill [3] published the first long-term result after surgical removal of a solitary hypernephroma metastasis in the lungs. The patient died of heart failure 23 years later. Alexander and Haight [2] presented a large series of patients for the first time in 1947. Kelly and Langston [17] were able to report on more than 100 published cases from the world literature in 1956. Since then, the pulmonary metastases of extrapulmonary primary tumors have been dealt with surgically to an increasing extent in parallel to the further development of the surgical therapy of bronchial carcinoma. Thomford et al. [41] already reported in 1965 on 205 patients operated on at the Mayo Clinic. Today, the estimated number of patients operated on for pulmonary metastases is about 10,000 all over the world [25].

With regard to the indication, there is still great uncertainty owing to the incomplete knowledge of the possibilities and limitations of surgery of pulmonary metastases and in view of the large degree of ignorance of the process of metastatic spreading, so that overtherapy and undertherapy are very close together [43].

Interdisciplinary Therapeutic Collaboration

Markedly improved survival rates after surgical treatment of pulmonary metastases in combination with an increasingly extended chemotherapy in some tumors have favored this trend towards an increase in surgery of pulmonary metastases. Thus the improvement of the possibility of chemotherapy led to an extension of the indications for sur-

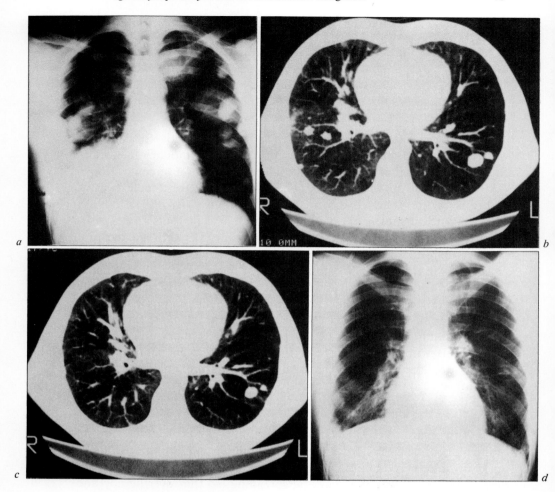

Fig. 1. Patient U.V., 21 years old, male. Testicular teratoma on the left, condition after left semicastration with retroperitoneal lymphadenectomy, 7/86. *a* Multiple pulmonary metastases on both sides, beta-HCG 155, alpha-fetoprotein over 400, 8/86. *b* CT during partial remission under chemotherapy (Einhorn scheme), 10/86. *c* CT after further remission at the end of chemotherapy, 1/87. *d* Partial remission with multiple residual metastases, beta-HCG and alpha-fetoprotein in the normal range, 2/87. Operation (resection of 24 metastases; histological examination shows that some of the metastases are still vital).

gery with regard to the various kinds of primary tumors as well as the numbers of metastases to be operated on. No longer only solitary metastases [2, 7], but also multiple metastases initially still localized unilaterally [41], and then also bilaterally [22, 29], as well as recurrent metastases [21] could now be treated by a rational combination of medical and surgical measures. It could be shown that the 5-year survival rates after resection of solitary and multiple metastases do not differ appreciably [22, 29, 45]. Constantly increasing new scientific knowledge gives rise to continuous changes in the boundary between locoregional surgical therapy and systemic chemotherapy. The attempts made with locoregional chemotherapy of pulmonary metastases so far have not yet been successful, in contrast, for example, to hepatic metastases of colorectal carcinomas. At present, surgical resection is probably the only potentially curative method of treatment of patients with pulmonary metastases [36]. Chemotherapy and possibly radiotherapy are to be considered in some forms of tumors, e. g. in osteosarcomas or rhabdomyosarcomas. However, as a rule manifest pulmonary metastases cannot be cured by chemotherapy. Pulmonary and lymph node metastases of testicular teratomas for which a very potent chemotherapy is available and for which surgery is to be regarded as adjuvant therapy constitute an exception (fig. 1).

In the diagnosis of a metastatic cancer condition, the visible metastasis found clinically will be the exception as compared to the metastasis which is not found and is not visible [19]. Micrometastases which cannot be diagnosed with the methods available to us today constitute the fundamental problem and the limiting parameter of metastasis surgery [37]. Since micrometastatic spreading is the domain of chemotherapy, further improvements in the results are conceivable by ameliorations to adjuvant chemotherapy. Moreover, it is evident that the removal of several or multiple metastases is meaningful, especially when an adjuvant chemotherapy is available, since in such cases the probability of micrometastatic spreading is very great. For tumors without available chemotherapy, such as hypernephromas or colorectal carcinomas, for example, it should be noted that solitary or few metastases can be removed with the objective of cure, whereas resection of several or multiple metastases is to be regarded as a prognostically palliative measure.

Resection of multiple metastases should be regarded predominantly as tumor reduction. A maximum tumor reduction leaving behind small tumor residues, e. g. on the large intrathoracic vessels, can be meaning-ful when a postoperative chemotherapy is possible. The tumor mass is of superordinate importance for the result of chemotherapy [8]. Both have a reciprocal relationship to each other. Thus, curability can still be attained by surgical tumor reduction after prior chemotherapy when healing is no longer possible by chemotherapy alone. On the other hand, this combined procedure can reduce the scale of the operation. To what extent the tumor reduction must be carried out, i. e. how much residual tumor may be left behind in order to attain a complete remis-sion on the basis of the subsequent chemotherapy, is so far still un-known for surgery of pulmonary metastases. We know from combined treatment of ovarian carcinomas that a reduction of remaining intra-peritoneal tumor masses to less than 1.5 cm diameter is of prognostic importance [32].

Principles of Metastasis Surgery

Theoretical principles concerning the indication for surgery of me-tastases derive from the types of metastases found by Walther [46] in 1948 and the cascade theory of metastatic spreading developed from these in 1976 by Bross and Blumenson [4]. Accordingly, tumor dissemi-nation follows pathways determined by the localization of the primary tumor and its venous or lymphatic drainage, and metastases are initially formed in the respective blood filters.

For the surgeon, caval and portal types of metastatic spreading with the lungs and liver as the first filter organs are of particular therapeutic importance. Generalized metastatic spreading of the tumor into the periphery only arises secondarily from the primary metastases in one or two organs of generalization.

The organs of generalization (mostly lungs and liver) are hence also designated as 'key organs'. It is suspected that a selection of tumor cells takes place in the formation of the first metastases. These tumor cells are capable of forming further metastases [11]. Eder [10] confirmed these rather theoretical concepts in autopsy material.

In knowledge of this cascade-like process of metastatic spreading, surgical reintervention with the objective of potential cure must take place in the stage of metastasis formation in the organ of generalization before onset of generalization. Treatment of metastases in the organ of generalization is thus a second key point in surgery of carcinomas and must be regarded in the same way in therapeutic terms as the primary tumor [37].

Diagnostic Problems

In most patients, the putative diagnosis 'pulmonary metastasis(es)' appears highly probable solely in view of the tumor history and the radiological criteria. The larger the number of nodules found scattered over both lungs, the more certain this is. Diagnosis of the tumor type becomes more difficult in all cases with solitary nodules. This may in principle involve a pulmonary metastasis, but a primary lung tumor or even a benign focus also appears to be possible. It is known from the literature that the probability of a solitary pulmonary nodule being a metastasis rises from less than 1% in patients with no history of tumors to more than 80% in cases with prior malignancy [48]. Cahan et al. [5] investigated this retrospectively and in a simplification formulated the following definition: as a rule, in patients with a known squamous epithelial carcinoma in their history, a newly occurring solitary nodule in the lungs is a new primary lung tumor. An adenocarcinoma known in the case history is with equal probability either a metastasis or a primary lung tumor. If the patient has previously had a sarcoma or a melanoma, the new pulmonary nodule is usually a metastasis. Finally, when there is a lymphoma in the anamnesis, it is mostly a new primary lung tumor.

In our own patients, on the basis of radiological findings we were able to make the primary putative diagnosis 'pulmonary metastasis(es)' in 94%, and in the remaining 6% this suspicion arose primarily from computer tomography and could then be confirmed in all cases by conventional X-rays. Altogether, a computer tomography of the lungs was carried out in only 211 patients (72%), owing to the fact that the period of observation extended back to 1972. Apart from the diagnosis of the kind of tumor, it is very important to know the number of metastases as precisely as possible in order to establish the indication for therapy and surgical operation which may have to be carried out.

The results show that several and indeed multiple metastases can be extirpated with the objective of cure, but a diffuse multiple metastatic spreading of pleuritis carcinomatosa constitutes a contraindication for surgical operation with the exception of diagnostic thoracotomy.

By means of conventional tomography of the lungs, additional information can be obtained on the presence and in particular on the number of possible metastases. At present, computer tomography is the most sensitive non-invasive method for detection of small intrapulmonary or pleural foci. Chang et al. [6] were able to show in a prospective study of 25 patients with 53 pulmonary metastases which were indeed resected that only 21 suspect nodules were detected in the scout view of the lungs, that almost twice as many nodules were found by additional conventional tomograms [38], and that finally computer tomography revealed 69 pulmonary nodules. The specificity thus decreases with higher sensitivity, i. e. of the nodules discovered by conventional X-rays 90% were indeed metastases, but only 66% in the conventional tomograms and only 45% in CT. Indeed, 15 metastases wer not detected preoperatively by any of the 3 methods, and the accuracy of the 3 methods was 36%, 47% and 58% respectively. Friedmann et al. [12] found the exact number of metastases using the 3 methods in 56%, 61% and 68% respectively in 24 patients with 51 pulmonary metastases the existence of which was later proved.

Since 1980, we therefore regularly require a preoperative computer tomogram. Especially in small pulmonary nodules and nodules of different generations, a preoperative CT is of great value not only with regard to maximum precision of preoperative diagnosis, but also because of a greater certainty that all metastases will be found intraoperatively. The appreciable uncertainty in the diagnosis of the exact number of metastases is also reflected in our own patients and has consequences for the surgical technique [44]. The same number of metastases as was diagnosed preoperatively was found intraoperatively in only 58% of our

Table I. Difference between preoperatively diagnosed and postoperatively verified number of metastases

Number of Metastases preoperative/postoperative		
Postoperative = preoperative	n = 177	58.2%
Postoperative > preoperative	n = 117	38.5%
Postoperative < preoperative	n = 10	3.3%

patients. On the other hand, more metastases were found intraoperatively in 39%, and fewer metastases were found intraoperatively in only 3% (table I).

Improvements are to be expected here from new techniques. In a study which is in progress at present, it is becoming apparent that much more exact preoperative determination of the number of metastases is possible using 'whole thorax tomograms' [42]. The large number of different primary tumors in surgery of pulmonary metastases makes it evident that preoperative staging must take into account the respective predilection site of metastatic spreading (e. g. bone, brain).

In principle, a sonographic or possibly a computer tomographic examination of the abdomen (especially of the liver and adrenals) must be part of this investigation. A local recurrence must always be ruled out.

If there is an unclear intra-abdominal finding (e. g. in the liver or adrenals), in lateral thoracotomy laparotomy can be carried out initially transdiaphragmatically and via an extension of the excision in median sternotomy. The operation is then continued or discontinued depending on the result of rapid-section histology. We proceeded in this way in 11% (n = 39) of cases.

Indications for Surgery of Metastases

The preconditions valid today for a potentially curative operation on metastases are summarized in table II. Before each operation, a check as to whether these preconditions have been fulfilled must be made. The primary tumor should have been radically resected and a local recurrence should be ruled out. Otherwise, it must be at least possible to remove completely the primary tumor or local recurrence immediately after resection of the metastases. On the basis of subtle diagnos-

Table II. Prerequisites for potentially curative resection of pulmonary metastases

1. Primary tumor treated curatively (treatable)
2. No extra-pulmonary metastatic sites demonstrable
3. Metastases resectable
4. Justifiable general and functional risk

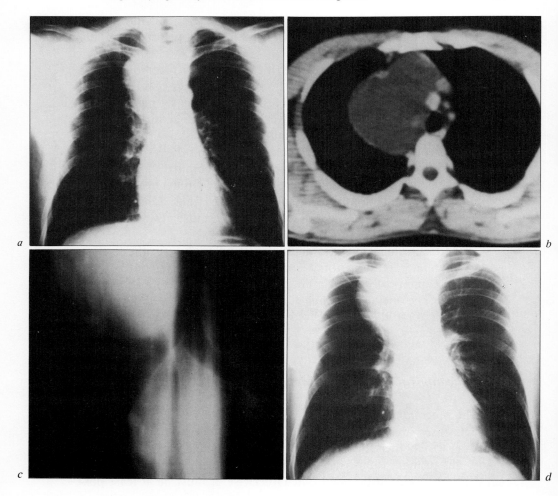

Fig. 2. Patient W. V., 27 years old, male. Testicular teratoma on the right, condition after right semicastration, 6/86, retroperitoneal lymphadenectomy, 12/86. *a* Large mediastinal lymph node metastases, beta-HCG 131, alpha-fetoprotein 310, simultaneously enlarged retroperitoneal lymph nodes, 6/86. *b* CT during chemotherapy (Einhorn scheme): large tumor in the anterior mediastinum and right paramediastinum, 10/86. *c* Hilus-filter layer shows a compression of the right upper lobe and the trachea by the mediastinal tumor, 2/87. *d* Despite chemotherapy, increase of mediastinal finding, beta-HCG and alpha-fetoprotein are once more in the normal range, 2/87. Surgery (radical extirpation of a largely necrotic tumor from lymph node packets with connective-tissue capsule).

tics, further distant metastases outside the lung should be ruled out, i. e. only an isolated metastasis in the lungs should be present. However, the question must remain open as to what extent the additional presence of even one extrapulmonary metastasis (e. g. in the liver or in the brain) constitutes a contraindication to resection of metastases. Valid appraisals on this will only be possible on the basis of future studies.

Simultaneous revision of several body cavities (e. g. of both lungs including the mediastinum and the abdomen in addition), allows simultaneous removal of pulmonary and extrapulmonary metastases, e. g. of hepatic or adrenal metastases [44]. In most cases several criteria are important for such a decision. At the present time, the removal of multiple-organ metastases is not by any means to be regarded as a recommended therapy and should be reserved for selected individual cases.

In principle, resection of metastases can only be potentially curative when there is macroscopic radicality. Local operability must hence be clarified preoperatively as far as possible. It is self-evident that the individual and absolute risk of surgery is to be appraised in comparison to the risk of the disease. Finally, a check must always be made to find out whether surgery is the sole form of therapy which is to be considered, or whether a potent nonsurgical form of therapy is available as an alternative.

A visible metastasis may be a first sign of a shooting-up of multiple metastases. We must hence initially wait for 8 weeks after the primary diagnosis and then carry out a fresh staging. If there is no indication of an exacerbation of the metastases after 8 weeks, we regard surgery as indicated. We believe that the danger of a possible 'overtreatment' is counteracted with this procedure.

However, the choice of the correct time in surgery of metastases has not been satisfactorily solved. Only if there is no furhter reduction in size or a fresh increase in size of the metastases under chemotherapy (fig. 2) can the operation be carried out immediately. On the other hand, if there is rapid progression of the condition under chemotherapy, surgical intervention is no longer indicated. If the preconditions for the resection of metastases (operation) are fulfilled, the following indications can be specified:

Solitary or few metastases. These are the classical indications for surgical therapy (e. g. hypernephroma), even when there are no possibilities of adjuvant therapy. In solitary pulmonary nodules, surgery is already indicated for reasons of differential diagnosis, since a nodule may correspond to a metastasis only with the probability of 80% even if there is a history of malignancy.

Multiple metastases are not a contraindication as long as it appears possible to remove all visible metastases preoperatively. It remains an open question at present as to the maximum number of metastases up to which surgery is still feasible. A better prognosis is to be expected in tumor forms which can receive preoperative and postoperative adjuvant chemotherapy (e. g. osteosarcoma, some soft-tissue sarcomas).

Solitary or occasional recurrent metastases can be operated on several times with the objective of cure [21] until the patients finally remain free of tumors. This phenomenon is observed above all in testicular teratoma and in sarcomas.

Resection for tumor reduction is only indicated in metastases sensitive to chemotherapy (e. g. testicular tumors, osteosarcoma, some soft-tissue sarcomas). This is based on the idea that there is a reciprocal relationship between tumor mass and the result of chemotherapy.

Residual metastases after chemotherapy are a further indication. They probably consist of tumor cell populations which do not respond at all or hardly respond to chemotherapy of the selected dosage or type. The residual foci frequently show a transformation from a mostly relatively undifferentiated primary tumor to highly differentiated and thus therapy-resistant cell populations. We established this indication several times in testicular teratomas. The further chemotherapeutic procedure is decided upon depending on the result of histological investigation.

Scar tissue after chemotherapy may be extirpated after complete remission of pulmonary metastases with critical consideration of the risk of surgery, since it is assumed that recurrences develop from these residual foci. Above all, testicular teratomas and osteosarcomas are involved here.

Elimination of complications due to metastases in terms of palliative criteria. This is indicated especially in pulmonary metastases infiltrating the chest wall accompanied by pain or impending or present tumor exulcerations which cannot be influenced in another way. Hemorrhages and tumor breakdown are also to be considered here.

Biopsy or diagnostic thoracotomy for the determination of receptors (e. g. breast cancer) and for the evaluation of the feasibility or efficiency of cytostatic therapy by viability tests.

Materials and Methods

In a retrospective analysis of operated patients with pulmonary metastases from the years 1972 to 1984, we determined the long-term results after resection of metastases and investigated the influence of potential prognostic factors for the probability of survival. In the observation period, our patients comprised 261 cases in whom a total of 295 operations had been carried out for pulmonary metastases. Twenty-nine patients thus had to be subjected to a total of 34 reoperations owing to development of fresh metastases. Since 9 patients were operated on consecutively via a lateral thoracotomy, the total number of 304 thoracotomies resulted (table III). One hundred and fifty-six patients (i. e. 60% of our patients) have died in the meantime.

The analysis of survival time relates to the total number of 261 patients. Of these, 54% were men and 46% were women. The average age was 45 years, the youngest patient operated on being 7 years old and the oldest patient 77 years old. The peak of the age distribution was between the 41st and 60th year of life (44% of our patients were within this age range). Twenty-eight percent were between 11 and 30 years old. This youngest patient group consisted almost exclusively of patients with metastases of osteosarcomas and testicular teratoma.

The primary tumors were 73% (n = 191) carcinomas and 27% (n = 70) sarcomas. Patients with breast cancer metastases and patients with testicular teratoma, hypernephroma and colorectal metastases constituted the largest single groups among the carcinomas (table IV). Among the sarcomas, the osteosarcomas were the largest single group and were contrasted with the group of soft-tissue sarcomas. In 8 patients who were operated on for one or several round foci and in whom a carcinoma metastasis was established histologically, the primary tumor remained undiscovered.

For the evaluation of the results of surgery on metastases, it is important to distinguish between potentially curative and noncurative operations, since the indication for metastasectomy should be established with the intention of potential cure.

However, the concept 'potentially curative' is to be appraised differently in surgery of metastases than in surgery of the primary tumor. Sixty-four operations in 63 patients were classified as noncurative, i. e. it was not possible in 24% of the patients to remove all visible and palpable tumor portions. Carcinomas and sarcomas did not differ in their relation (table V). The most frequent reason (table VI) for a noncurative operation was

Table III. Frequencies of re-thoracotomy in surgery of metastases of the lungs

Number of operations per patient

232 patients	1× = 232	
25 patients	2× = 50	29 patients,
3 patients	3× = 9	34 reoperations
1 patient	4× = 4	

261 patients → 295 operations (304 thoracotomies)

Table IV. Primary tumor localizations of 261 patients operated on for pulmonary metastases

Carcinomas (n = 191)	
Caval type of metastases (n = 157)	
Breast	34
Female genitals	
Cervix	12
Corpus	1
Vagina	1
Ovary	3
Male genitals	
Testis	32
Prostate	1
Kidney and bladder	
Hypernephroma	32
Wilms'	3
Bladder	4
Head and neck	
Larynx	1
Tonsil	1
Hypopharynx	1
Tongue	2
Parotid	2
Chest	
Lung	10
Heart	1
Thymus	1
Other	
Adrenal	2
Thyroid	3
Liver	1
Extragonad. teratoma	1
Melanoma	8
Portal type of metastases (n = 26)	
Colorectal	
Colon	15
Rectum	10
Other	
Pancreas	1
Primary site unknown (n = 8)	

Table IV. Continued

Sarcomas (n = 70)	
Osteosarcoma	28
Soft-tissue sarcomas	
Synovialsarcoma	14
Fibrosarcoma	10
Rhabdomyosarcoma	4
Leiomyosarcoma	3
Haemangiopericytoma	2
Liposarcoma	1
Other	
Ewing's sarcoma	4
Chodronsarcoma	3
Reticulosarcoma	1

Table V. Number of noncurative operations (in % of all operations) in relation to tumor type and primary tumor

	n	%
Carcinomas	(44/203)	21.7%
Caval type	(37/172)	21.5%
Portal type	(7/ 31)	22.6%
Sarcomas	(20/ 92)	21.7%
Osteosarcoma	(13/ 41)	31.7%
Other	(7/ 51)	13.7%
Total	(64/295)	21.7%

the multiple metastatic spreading of mainly very tiny metastases which were then usually not resectable and which were surprisingly discovered intraoperatively. The next largest group of patients were those with a large tumor mass which was mostly already known preoperatively and in whom a complete resection was no longer possible owing to the extent of the tumor. The thoracotomies performed for purely diagnostic reasons in already visible multiple metastases for the purpose of histological verification or appraisal of the possibilities or efficiency of chemotherapy and for determination of receptors (e. g. in breast cancer) were naturally appraised as noncurative. The same applies to resections of metastases in an unknown primary tumor.

Table VI. Main criteria for classification as noncurative operations

	n
1. Surprising multiple metastases	25
2. Tumor spreading (local inoperability)	18
3. Primary tumor cannot be located	3
4. Diagnostic thoracotomy (preoperative multiple metastases unknown)	18
Total	64

The calculation of the probabilities of survival was carried out according to the statistical model of Kaplan and Meier [16]. To test the prognostic relevance of the different parameters, the log-rank test [33] was employed to analyse the survival curves with censored data. The date set for the evaluation was April 30th, 1986. The observation period for all patients was thus at least 1.3 years, so long as they had not died beforehand.

Long-Term Results

The overall survival rates of the 261 paients were 69% after 1 year, 41% after 3 years and 32% after 5 years (fig. 3) with a median survival of 24.7 months. If a distinction is made between patients with potentially curative and noncurative resection there is, as expected, a highly significant difference: the probability of 5-year survival in the patients with the potentially curative resection is 38% (fig. 4). This 38% constitutes the actual overall result of metastasis surgery with a median survival time of 31 months. Of the patients with noncurative resection, 16% still survive after 5 years, and the median survival is 13.7 months. This is explained by the maximum tumor reduction with subsequent chemotherapy carried out in many cases. Apart from this, it is shown that the spontaneous course is not to be neglected in the consideration of the long-term results.

The following results are related exclusively to the group of patients with a potentially curative operation.

Whereas the comparison of the tumor classes carcinomas and sarcomas did not reveal any significant difference in the survival times, a significant (p = 0.048) advantage for the cavally metastasizing carcino-

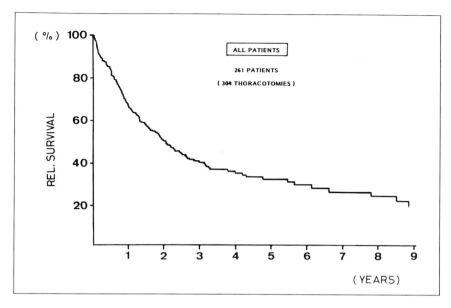

Fig. 3. Probabilities of survival of all patients with a potentially curative and non-curative resection for pulmonary metastases.

mas with a 5-year actuarial survival of 42% and a median survival of 39 months as compared to 37% and 23 months median survival were shown after differentiation of the carcinomas into caval and portal type of metastatic spreading. With the inclusion of sarcomas with a 5-year actuarial survival of 28% and 18 months median survival, there remains a significant difference between the tumor groups (fig. 5).

There is no statistically significant difference between the group of sarcomas and the group of carcinomas of portal type. Accordingly, the prognosis for carcinomas of caval type is very much better than that of sarcomas (p = 0.039).

Upon separate consideration of the largest groups of primary tumors, a significant difference is found (fig. 6). By far the best prognosis is shown in the patients after resection of metastases of testicular teratoma with a 5-year actuarial survival of 71%. No patients die 3 years after surgery. The poorest 5-year actuarial survival is shown by the colorectal carcinomas, which nevertheless display 37% and a median survival of

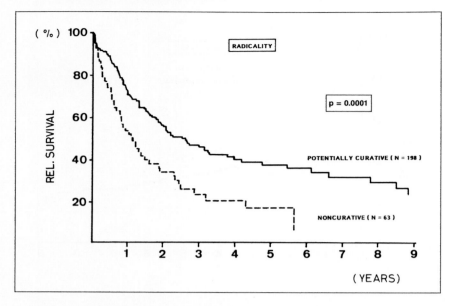

Fig. 4. Probabilities of survival depending on the radicality of the operation.

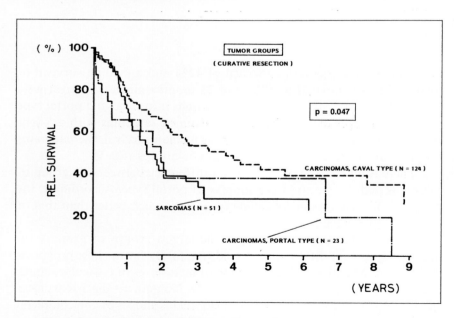

Fig. 5. Probabilities of survival depending on the tumor group.

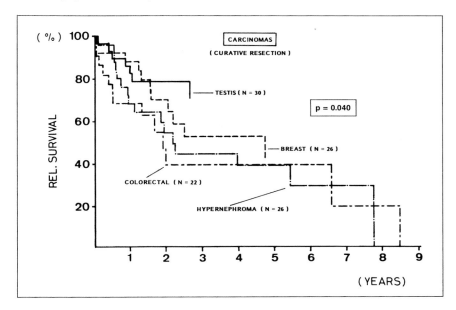

Fig. 6. Probabilities of survival of carcinomas depending on the primary tumor localization.

23 months as well as hypernephromas with 38% and a median survival of 26 months. The breast cancer survival rates are very much higher; of these, 42% survive for 5 years and the median survival is 57 months.

In the smaller primary tumor groups which still allow statistical analysis, a 5-year actuarial survival of 50% was found in the carcinomas of the head and neck region as well as in cervical carcinomas. The prognosis of the melanoma patients, 25% of whom were still alive after 3 years, but none of whom was alive after 5 years, was very much poorer.

In the poorer sarcoma group, the soft-tissue sarcoma with a 5-year actuarial survival of 35% and a median survival of 22 months had better results than the osteosarcomas with a 3-year actuarial survival of 24% and a median survival of 16 months. The difference between the soft-tissue and osteosarcomas is not significant, however.

The disease-free interval between operation on the primary tumor and occurrence of pulmonary metastases constitutes a crucial prognostic criterion. There are highly significant differences, with a threshold value at 3 years (fig. 7). Patients with a shorter interval have a probabili-

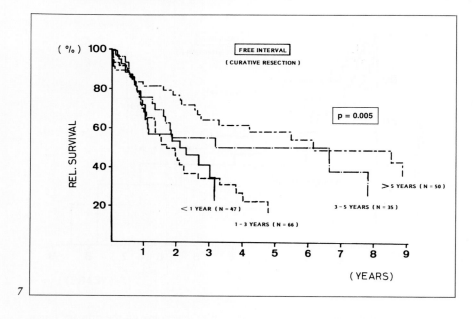

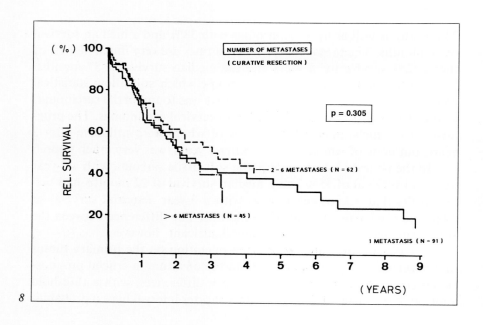

ty of 17% of surviving for 5 years and a median survival of 20 months, whereas the corresponding values with a larger interval were 50% with a median survival time of 37 months. If the metastases occurred more than 5 years after operation on the primary tumor, 58% still survived for 5 years with a median survival time of 73 months. Early metastatic spreading is thus a poor prognostic sign even in complete metastasis resection.

Surprisingly, we did not find any appreciable influence of the number of metastases on the prognosis amongst the patients with curative surgery (fig. 8). It is accordingly immaterial how many metastases are removed, provided that the surgeon succeeds in completely removing all visible and palpable metastases. This becomes evident when the group of patients not operated on curatively is included in this consideration. A significant difference (p = 0.023) is then found between the patients with fewer than 6 metastases and those with more metastases. The 5-year actuarial survivals are 40% as compared to 18%, and there is also a marked difference between the median survival of 32 as opposed to 18 months. This is explained by the fact that the vast majority of patients with noncurative surgery had more than 6 metastases. The example illustrates that a subdivision into curatively and noncuratively operated patients is important in analyzing the results of metastasis surgery.

In accordance with the results for the number of metastases, we still did not find any difference in the patients with curative resection between metastatic infiltration of one or both lungs.

In consideration of all primary tumors, the metastasis size does not have any statistical influence on the prognosis (fig. 9). In separate analyses of the groups of carcinomas of caval and portal type of metastatic spreading, this result is confirmed. On the other hand, in the sarcomas a highly significant difference is found between metastases with a diameter of more than 3 cm and those of up to 3 cm (fig. 10). When the metastases were smaller, the 5-year actuarial survival was 37% with a

Fig. 7. Probabilities of survival depending on the disease-free interval (macroscopic radical metastasis resection).

Fig. 8. Probabilities of survival depending on the number of resected metastases (radical metastasis resection).

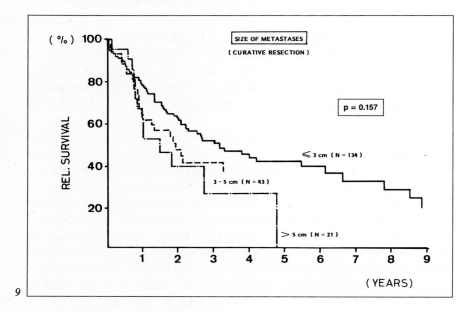

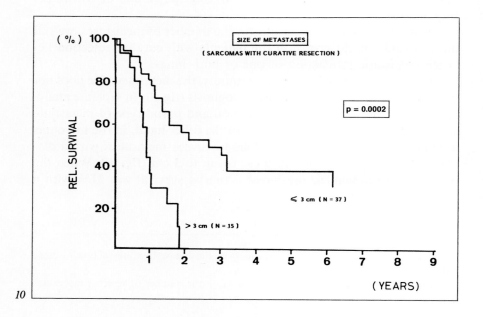

median survival of 31 months. On the other hand, no patient with large metastases survived for 3 years, and for this group the median survival was only 11 months.

The comparison of the resection technique applied shows a significant difference between the probabilities of survival (fig. 11). For the atypical resections, segment resections and enucleations, the 5-year actuarial survival was 44% with a median survival of 50 months, as compared to 30% for lobectomy with a median survival of 25 months. After performance of bilobectomy or pneumonectomy owing to a central localization of metastases or a large tumor mass, no patient survived for as long as 5 years, and the median survival was merely 9 months.

Accordingly, preoperative direct or indirect bronchoscopic detection of the tumor (n = 44) as far as the segmental branches of the bronchus did not have any significant effect on the probability of survival (fig. 12), since the prognostically unfavorable bilobectomies and pneumonectomies could be avoided in 36% by bronchoplastic or angioplastic operations (fig. 13). Fifty-seven percent of all plastic techniques (n = 28) were carried out after bronchoscopic tumor detection. A comparison of the 23 bronchoplastic or angioplastic extended resections carried out with the objective of cure with standard resections, however, reveals a highly significant difference: only 11% of patients with plastic extension of the operation reach the 3-year survival limit and no patient survives for 5 years, the median survival being 11.6 months. On the other hand, 40.3% of patients survived for 5 years after standard resection techniques, with a median survival of 35.5 months.

The histological detection of a metastatic intrapulmonary or mediastinal lymph node infiltration also did not result in any deterioration of the prognosis (fig. 14). Unfortunately, there is no possibility so far of distinguishing with certainty between lymph node metastatic spreading into the lungs (e. g. testicular teratoma) or from the lungs. The latter would have to be at the beginning of an incipient generalization.

Fig. 9. Probabilities of survival in relation to the size of the resected metastases (all patients with a potentially curative resection).

Fig. 10. Probabilities of survival of the patients with metastases of sarcomas in relation to the size of the resected metastases.

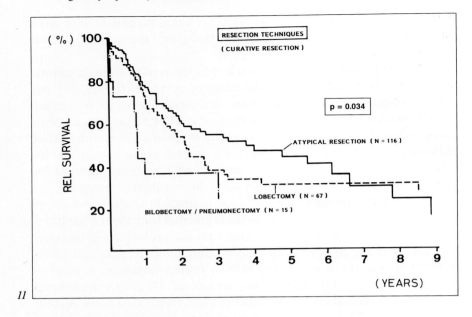

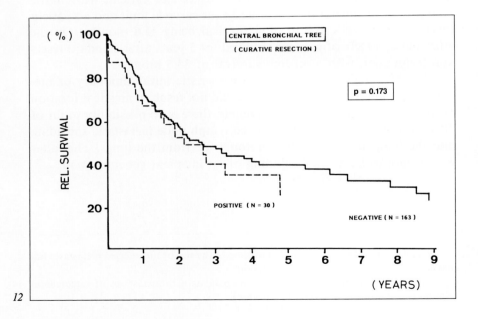

Critical Considerations, Conclusion and Outlook

Today, surgical treatment of pulmonary metastases is an established technique in the interdisciplinary concept of oncological therapy. Our own overall result of a 5-year actuarial survival of 32% corresponds to the international standard (table VII).

Unfortunately, data are only very rarely provided as to whether the operations were curative or noncurative. The 5-year actuarial survival times in 76% of the patients with potentially curative macroscopically radial operations was 38% for all organ tumors. Takita [39] and Merlier [26] confirmed this result with 34% and 33% actuarial survivals after a potentially curative operation. These figures are comparable with the results after resection of other nonmetastasizing tumors and correspond to those of primary bronchial carcinoma in stages I and II of our patients [28].

Determination of prognostic factors constitutes the attempt to work out patient groups which have the greatest proportion of metastasis operations. In particular the tumor doubling time with a limit at about 40 days appears to be a substantiated criterion [34, 37, 39]. Other factors are discussed controversially [34, 39], and statements by the same authors are revised again after longer periods of observation [39, 40], so that generally valid statements cannot yet be made. Nevertheless, the disease-free interval, the number of metastases, the lymph node involvement, the size of the metastases and in particular the resectability appear to be of prognostic significance [34, 39]. Putnam [34] found that the combination of several significant single factors was the best indicator for the long-term postoperative prognosis.

Our analysis was able to show (table VIII) that complete resection of all visible and palpable metastases is decisive for the result. Accordingly, the number of metastases is of subordinate significance, provided it does not limit the resectability, i. e. radicality. For the group of curatively resected patients, the disease-free interval with a limit at 3 years

Fig. 11. Probabilities of survival in relation to the respective resection technique applied.

Fig. 12. Probabilities of survival in relation to the bronchoscopic finding (visible tumor extending into the subsegmental ramifications).

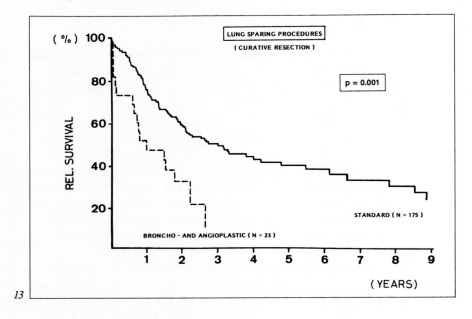

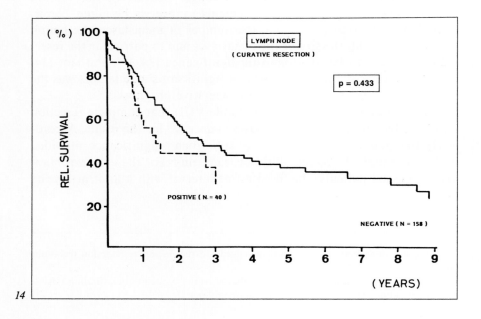

Table VII. Collected statistics of the 5-year actuarial survival times after resection of pulmonary metastases (literature review)

Author	Year	n	Survivors (n)	%
Thomford et al. [41]	1965	205	62	30
McCormack [23]	1978	215	45	21
Wilkins [49]	1978	140	43	31
Gall et al. [13]	1979	67	28	42
Morrow et al. [31]	1980	167	48	29
Marks et al. [20]	1981	90	30	33
Metzger et al. [27]	1981	64	22	35
Shepherd [28]	1982	47	7	15
Wright et al. [51]	1982	140	36	26
Head [15]	1983	205	65	32
Mountain et al. [30]	1984	443	155	35
Vogt-Moykopf et al. [45]*	1986	261	84	32
12 authors		2,044	625	31

* Overall result for all patients with potentially curative as well as noncurative operations

Table VIII. Significance of prognostic factors for the probability of survival

Prognostic factors	
Significant	*Nonsignificant*
Radicality	Tumor class
Route of metastatic spreading	Number of metastases
Type of primary tumor	Unilateral/bilateral
Disease-free interval	Involvement of lymph nodes
Size of metastases	Involvement of the central bronchial
Resection technique	tree

Fig. 13. Probabilities of survival in relation to a bronchoplastic or angioplastic extension of the resection.

Fig. 14. Probabilities of survival in relation to metastatic lymph node infiltration.

Table IX. Results of surgery on metastases of the lungs depending on the primary tumor localization

Primary tumor	n	Survival time		
		3 years (%)	5 years (%)	median (mos.)
Osteosarcoma	18	24	—	16
Soft-tissue sarcoma	33	43	35	22
Testis teratoma	29	71	—	—
Hypernephroma	25	44	38	26
Breast	26	52	42	57
Cervix	10	50	50	25
Colorectal	22	39	37	23
Head and neck	7	80	50	50
Melanoma	6	25	0	11

is an unequivocal prognostic criterion. At least in the carcinomas, the primary tumor type and the type of metastatic spreading is of great importance. The cavally metastasizing carcinomas had the best prognosis with a probability of 5-year survival of 42%. This corresponds to the cascade theory of metastatic spreading [4], according to which pulmonary metastases with the liver as the first organ of generalization are to be rated as having a poorer prognosis than that of tumors in which the lungs are the first organ of generalization. The excellent result for testicular teratomas, for which a probability of 5-year survival cannot be specified because no patients die after the third year, points to the importance of an adequate chemotherapy, the presence of which has a favorable influence on the course and can extend the indication. On the other hand, the results in our own patients are if anything sobering in osteocarcinoma sensitive to chemotherapy and do not correspond to the good results of other authors [21, 37]. In agreement with the results of almost all authors [30, 36], on the other hand, our few patients with melanoma metastases also had a very poor prognosis, and the indication for surgery will have to be established only with very great reserve in the future under current conditions (table IX). With a limit of 3 cm, the size of metastases so far only appears to be of significance in sarcomas. The principle of resection in surgery of metastases which conserves as much parenchyma as possible could be confirmed by the best long-term results after smaller atypical and segment resections with adequate radicality.

Results of surgery of metastases can be compared only with very great difficulty (table VII), since an urgently required staging is so far not available, and differences in strictness in establishment of the indication in highly heterogenous patient groups influence the results. Primary tumor localizations, primary therapy, histology and criteria of malignancy, grading of the primary tumors, preoperative and postoperative treatment as well as establishment of the indication and surgical therapy are all nonuniform, which underscores the dilemma in the appraisal of the results of treatment. Although only the comparison with the spontaneous course of the disease can reveal the value of a therapy, little is known about the spontaneous course of pulmonary metastases in relation to the different primary tumors. The good results after resection of metastases in breast cancer (table IX), which are confirmed in the literature [24, 49, 51] point in this direction. It is possible that patients who fulfill the criteria for surgical intervention constitute a strict selection of patients who already have a relatively good chance of surviving for 5 years anyway.

Aberg et al. [1] could not find any significant difference between operated patients and a control group with solitary pulmonary metastases. They call for a 10-year observation period for appraisal, since many patients still die of their cancer condition after 5 years. Other than in surgery of the primary tumor, the 10-year limit appears to be more relevant and more honest in its informational weight as a criterion of healing in surgery on metastases.

Patients who survived for 5 years after resection of metastases are frequently not free of tumors. In our own patients, 29 patients with a survival time of at least 5 years could already be observed so far. Of these, 7 died later. The cause of death was tumor-dependent in 5 patients, and 2 patients were free of tumors up to their death. Of the 22 patients still alive at the time of evaluation, 13 are so far still free of tumors.

Larger numbers of patient and longer periods of observation will enable relevant appraisals on this in the future. In particular, one must wait until relevant appraisals on the probability of survival for 10 years can be made for the first time on the basis of a larger number of patients. Up to the present time, we have not been able to obtain any valid data on this. However, it does not appear to be the case that surgery of metastases in the lungs and also in the liver is to be regarded as palliative from the start. Moreover, it must always be considered precisely in surgery of metastases that besides healing, the meaningful and possibly long-term prolongation of life may constitute a second goal of therapy which may be very valuable for the patient in the individual case.

With regard to life expectancy, healing and palliative treatment may indeed be identical in the extreme case [37]. The significant difference in the course between patients with potentially curative and noncurative operation indicates that radical resection of metastases at least has a marked life-prolonging effect.

Our own prognostic factors and those reported in the literature indicate that staging of pulmonary metastases may be possible in the future. It is likely to be a precondition for comparison of literature data and more precise establishment of the indication. However, it is exceedingly complicated to formulate such a staging in view of the large number of different primary tumors. At present, a satisfactory suggestion is not yet available which might do justice to the complexity of therapy in pulmonary metastases. For the time being, a series of prognostic factors should be considered in establishing the indication for surgery and should help to reduce the risk of undertherapy or overtherapy. The extent to which they can be crucial for the correct decision in the individual case must remain open. However, knowledge of these factors may influence the decision, especially in borderline cases. More sophisticated possibilities of chemotherapy and a more certain establishment of the indication will be able to improve further the encouraging results of metastasis surgery in the multimodal therapy concept.

References

1   Aberg, T.; Malmberg, K.-A.; Nilsson, B.; Nou, E.: The effect of metastasectomy: fact or fiction. Ann. thor. Surg. *30:* 378–384 (1980).
2   Alexander, J.; Haight, C.: Pulmonary resection for solitary metastatic sarcomas and carcinomas. Surgery Gynec. Obstet. *85:* 129–146 (1947).
3   Barney, J. D.; Churchill, E. J.: Adenocarcinoma of the kidney with metastases to the lung: cured by nephrectomy and lobectomy. J. Urol. (Baltimore) *42:* 269–276 (1939).
4   Bross, I. D. J.; Blumenson, L. E.: Metastatic sites that produce generalized cancer: identification and kinetics of generalizing sites; in: Weiss, Fundamental aspects of metastasis, pp. 359–375 (North-Holland, Amsterdam, New York 1976).

5   Cahan, W. C.; Castro, E. B.; Hajdu, S. I.: The significance of a solitary lung shadow in patients with colon carcinoma. Cancer *33:* 414–421 (1974).

6   Chang, A. E.; Schaner, E. G.; Conkle, A. M.: Evaluation of computed tomography in the detection of pulmonary metastases. Cancer *43:* 913–916 (1972).

7   Choksi, L. B.; Takita, H.; Vincent, R. G.: The surgical management of solitary pulmonary metastases. Surgery Gynec. Obstet. *134:* 479–482 (1972).

8   De Vita, V. T., Jr.: The relationship between tumor mass and resistance to chemotherapy. Cancer *51:* 1209–1220 (1983).

9   Divis, G.: Ein Beitrag zur operativen Behandlung der Lungengeschwülste. Acta chir. scand. *62:* 329–341 (1927).

10   Eder, M.: Die Metastasierung: Fakten und Probleme aus immunpathologischer Sicht. Verk. Dt. Ges. Path., vol. 68, pp. 1–11 (Fischer, Stuttgart, New York 1984).

11   Fidler, I. J.; Hart, J. R.: The origin of metastatic heterogenity in tumors. Eur. J. Cancer *17:* 487–494 (1981).

12   Friedmann, G.; Bohndorf, K.; Krüger, J.: Radiology of pulmonary metastases: comparison of imaging techniques with operative findings. Thorac. Cardiovasc. Surg. *34:* 120–124 (1986).

13   Gall, F. P.; Mühe, E.; Angermann, B.: Chirurgische Behandlung von Lungenmetastasen. Dt. med. Wschr. *104:* 835–837 (1979).

14   Gilbert, H. A.; Kagan, A. R.: Metastases: incidence, detection and evaluation without histological confirmation; in Weiss, Fundamental aspects of metastasis, pp. 315–405 (North-Holland, Amsterdam, Oxford 1976).

15   Head, J. M.: Surgery of pulmonary metastases; in Choi, Grillo. Thoracic oncology, pp. 359–365 (Raven, New York, 1983).

16   Kaplan, E. L.; Meier, P.: Non-parametric estimation from incomplete observation. J. Am. Statist. Assoc. *53:* 457–481 (1958).

17   Kelly, C. R.; Langston, H. T.: The treatment of metastatic pulmonary malignancy. J. thorac. Surg. *316:* 298–315 (1956).

18   Krönlein, E.: Über Lungenchirurgie. Berl. klin. Wschr. *9:* 129–136 (1884).

19   Liebig, S., Gabler, A.: Problematik und Wert der Stadieneinteilung für die Behandlung intrathorakaler Tumoren. Prax. Pneumol. *35:* 843–850 (1981).

20   Marks, P.; Ferrag, M. Z.; Ashraf, H.: Rationales for the surgical treatment of pulmonary metastases. Thorax *36:* 679–682 (1981).

21   Martini, N.; Huvos, A. G.; Mike, V. et al.: Multiple pulmonary resections in the treatment of osteogenic sarcoma. Ann. thor. Surg. *12:* 271–280 (1971).

22   Martini, N.; Bains, M. S.; Huvos, A. G.; Beattie, E. J.: Surgical treatment of metastatic sarcoma of the lung. Surg. Clins. N. Am. *54:* 841–848 (1974).

23   McCormack, P. M.: Surgical treatment of pulmonary metastases: Memorial Hospital Experience; in Weiss, Gilbert, Pulmonary metastases, pp. 260–270 (Martinus Nijhoff, The Hague, Boston, London 1978).

24   McCormack, P. M.; Martini, N.: The changing role of surgery for pulmonary metastases. Ann. thor. Surg. *28:* 139–144 (1979).

25   Merkle, N. M.; Meyer, G.; Bülzebruck, H.: Operative Behandlung von Lungenmetastasen; in Schildberg, pp. 191–206. Chirurgische Behandlung von Tumormetastasen (Bibliomed, Melsungen 1987).

26   Merlier, M.; Silbert, D.; Regnand, J. F.: Chirurgie à visée curative des metastases pulmonaires. Presse méd. *37:* 1907–1908 (1985).

27 Metzger, U.; Uhlschmid, G.; Largiader, F.: Die heutige Stellung der Chirurgie in der Behandlung von Lungenmetastasen. Schweiz. med. Wschr. *111:* 1303–1306 (1981).

28 Meyer, G.; Merkle, N. M.; Vogt-Moykopf, I.: Chirurgische Therapie des Bronchialkarzinoms. Münch. med. Wschr. *128:* 141–146 (1986).

29 Morton, D. L.; Joseph, W. L.; Ketcham, A. S.: Surgical resection and adjunctive immunotherapy for selected patients with multiple pulmonary metastases. Ann. Surg. *178:* 360–366 (1973).

30 Mountain, C. F.; McMurtrey, M. J.; Hermes, K. E.: Surgery for pulmonary metastasis: a 20-year experience. Ann. thor. Surg. *38:* 323–330 (1984).

31 Morrow, C. E.; Vassilopoulos, P. P.; Grage, T. B.: Surgical resection for metastatic neoplasms of the lung: experience at the University of Minnesota Hospitals. Cancer *45:* 2981–2985 (1980).

32 Osieka, R.; Schmidt, C. G.: Kombinierte onkologische Therapiekonzepte. Arch. klin. Chir. *361:* 513–518 (1983).

33 Peto, R.; Peto, J.: Asymptotically efficient rand invariant test procedures. J. Roy. Statist. Soc. A *135:* 185–206 (1972).

34 Putnam, J. B.; Roth, J. A.; Vescey, M. N. et al.: Analysis of prognostic factors in patients undergoing resection of pulmonary metastases from soft tissue sarcomas. J. thorac. cardiovasc. Surg. *87:* 260–268 (1984).

35 Röpke, E.: Zentbl. Univ. *64:* 803 (1937).

36 Roth, J. A.: Treatment of metastatic cancer to lung; in De Vita, Hellmann, Rosenberg, Cancer – Principles and Practice of Oncology, vol. 2, 2nd ed., pp. 2104–2117 (Lippincott, Philadelphia 1985).

37 Schildberg, F. W.; Meyer, G.; Wenk, H.: Der Stellenwert der Chirurgie bei der Therapie von Tumormetastasen; in Eigler, Peiper, Schildberg et al., Stand und Gegenstand der chirurgischen Forschung, pp. 457–487 (Springer, Berlin, Heidelberg, New York 1986).

38 Shepherd, M. P.: Thoracic metastases. Thorax *37:* 366–370 (1982).

39 Takita, H.; Edgerton, F.; Kakakousis, C. et al.: Surgical management of metastases to the lung. Surgery Gynec. Obstet. *152:* 191–194 (1981).

40 Takita, H.; Edgerton, F.; Merrin, C. et al.: Management of multiple lung metastases. J. surg. Oncol. *12:* 199–205 (1979).

41 Thomford, N. R.; Woolner, L. B.; Clagett, O. T.: The surgical treatment of metastatic tumors in the lungs. J. thorac. cardiovasc. Surg. *49:* 357–363 (1965).

42 Tuengerthal, S.: Persönliche Mitteilung (1978).

43 Vogt-Moykopf, I.; Meyer, G.; Bülzebruck, H.: Lungenmetastasen – Therapieindikation und chirurgische Technik. Münch. med. Wschr. *128:* 295–300 (1986).

44 Vogt-Moykopf, I.; Meyer, G.: Surgical technique in operations on pulmonary metastases. Thorac. cardiovasc. Surg. *34:* 125–132 (1986).

45 Vogt-Moykopf, I.; Meyer, G.; Merkle, N. M. et al.: Late results of surgical treatment of pulmonary metastases. Thorac. cardiovasc. Surg. *34:* 143–148 (1986).

46 Walther, H. E.: Krebsmetastasen (Schweiz, Basel 1948).

47 Weinlechner: Wien. med. Wschr. Nr. 20 + 21 (1882).

48 Weiss, L.; Gilbert, H. A.: Pulmonary metastases, pp. 142–167 (Hell, Boston 1978).

49 Wilkins, E. J.: The status of pulmonary resection of metastases: experience at Massachusetts General Hospital; in Weiss, Gilbert, Pulmonary metastases pp. 271–281 (Martinus Nijhoff, The Hague, Boston, London 1978).

50   Willis, R. A.: Pathology of tumors, p. 175 (Appleton-Century Crafts, London 1967).

51   Wright, J. O.; Brandt, B.; Ehrenhaft, J. L.: Results of pulmonary resection for metastatic lesions. J. thorac. cardiovasc. Surg. *83:* 94–99 (1982).

Prof. Dr. I. Vogt-Moykopf, Chirurgische Abteilung, Thoraxklinik der LVA Baden, Krankenhaus Rohrbach, Amalienstraße 5, D-6900 Heidelberg (FRG)

Contr. Oncol., vol. 30, pp. 108–131 (Karger, Basel 1988)

Surgical Strategy and Technique in Thoracotomy and Resection of Pulmonary Metastases

I. Vogt-Moykopf, G. Meyer, M. Langsdorf

Surgical Department, Hospital for Thoracic Diseases, Rohrbach Hospital, Heidelberg, FRG

Introduction

Specific features of tumor biology give rise to a series of particular demands on thoracic surgeons in carrying out resection of pulmonary metastases. This necessitates the development of new surgical strategies and operation techniques. In recent years, efforts have been concentrated in particular on establishing an optimal approach in thoracic surgical operations of metastases. This is a problem in its own right, since multiple and bilaterally localized metastases have also been subjected increasingly to resection treatment since the 1970s. An important new development in surgery of metastases was the introduction of median sternotomy with opening of both pleural cavities and the mediastinum from the front. This was first recommended by Takita [7] in 1977 on the basis of his own experience in a large number of patients. Using this approach, he removed up to 56 metastases on both sides in one session.

Special Surgically Relevant Features of Metastatic Spreading in the Lungs

Table I summarizes the features which should be taken into consideration in the choice of the surgical procedure. In our patients, bilateral metastatic spreading was present in 36% of cases, and in 27% of patients with known involvement only on one side preoperatively, metastases were also found intraoperatively in the contralateral lung. The number of metastases detected intraoperatively corresponded to that

Table I. Special features of pulmonary metastases with their technical relevance

1. Bilateral metastases
2. Uncertain diagnosis

⟶   Median thoracotomy as approach

3. Tendency to recurrence
4. Multiple metastases
5. Chemotherapy

⟶   Parenchyma-conserving resections

diagnosed preoperatively in only 58% of our patients, whereas more metastases were found intraoperatively in 39% and fewer metastases in only 3%. In agreement with other authors [1, 2], even with computer tomography performed preoperatively on principle as the most sensitive method available at present for detecting small intrapulmonary or pleural foci, about 30−40% of the metastases later found intraoperatively thus remain undiscovered up to operation.

Fifteen percent of our patients were operated on at least once because of metastatic recurrence. Multiple operations and recurrences are not uncommon. Solitary metastases were present in only 37% of the operations. In the majority, several to multiple metastases were found. However, only a small proportion of the multiple metastases found in 28% could be subjected to resection treatment with the aim of potential cure. For the long-term result, the number of resected metastases is less decisive, provided that they are technically operable and all visible or palpable metastases can be removed completely [8]. With regard to the long-term results, however, it must for the moment remain an open question as to the number of metastases up to which surgery is still appropriate. A better prognosis is to be expected in those forms of tumors which are susceptible to preoperative and postoperative adjuvant chemotherapy.

In view of the known facts confirmed in the international literature, median thoracotomy is to be recommended as the approach of first choice. With sufficient radicality, it must be aimed for as the resection technique conserving the most parenchyma.

The Value of Lateral Thoracotomy

In principle, posterolateral thoracotomy affords the best overview of the anterior and posterior part of the respective hemithorax, but has the disadvantage of only opening up for exploration the unilaterial hemithorax with its corresponding mediastinal part, and thus only enabling a unilateral procedure. Metastatic spreading on the opposite side not discovered preoperatively will thus remain concealed. Moreover, false appraisals of resectability may arise when, for example, all visible and palpable metastases on the one side are removed radically, but locally inoperable conditions are found later on the opposite side.

This disadvantage is also present in simultaneous bilateral thoracotomy. However, this has the advantage of being able to remove all metastases in one session and thus entails less psychological stress for the patient. In principle, anterior thoracotomy carried out in the supine position with the possibility of extension by transverse sternotomy or lateral thoracotomy on both sides may be considered. However, both procedures have serious disadvantages such as difficult access to the posterior parts of the lung and mediastinum, intraoperative repositioning or the very great surgical trauma for the patient.

Bilateral two-session lateral thoracotomy has the disadvantage of a double subjective stress for the patient as well as the doubled risk of surgery. In addition, there is the danger of a secondary inoperable situation already referred to in bilateral metastases owing to the lack of an overall scout view.

Unilateral single-session lateral thoracotomy remains indicated in 'definitive' unilateral tumors which are large or which infiltrate the posterior mediastinum. The approach via a lateral thoracotomy is also recommended in large-area infiltrations of the chest wall in which surgery of metastases can usually only be carried out on a palliative basis. Furthermore, an appreciably restricted respiratory reserve may favor the less stressful unilateral operation via a lateral thoracotomy, although it must always be considered in such cases that the certain radicality which is the objective of any operation on metastases is never assured [8].

The Advantages of Median Thoracotomy

Since 1981, we have chosen median sternotomy as the route of approach in increasing numbers of cases of surgery on pulmonary metastases. This is today our regular approach and was carried out 92 times by 1984 (fig. 1, table II). It enables simultaneous bilateral exploration or resection on the pleural membranes, and if necessary on the chest wall as well as both lungs and the entire mediastinum. Moreover, it affords the advantage of being readily able to prolong incision of

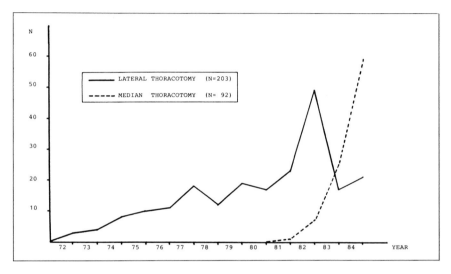

Fig. 1. Decrease in number of lateral thoracotomies and increase in number of median thoracotomies as an approach in surgery of pulmonary metastases.

Table II. Approaches in operations performed for pulmonary metastases

Thoracotomies	n	%
Posterolateral	152	51.5
Median	91	30.8
Posterior	27	9.2
Anterior	10	3.4
Posterolateral simultaneously on both sides	2	0.7
Posterolateral 2 sessions on both sides	9	3.1
Posterolateral double	3	1.0
Median and lateral	1	0.3
Total	295	100

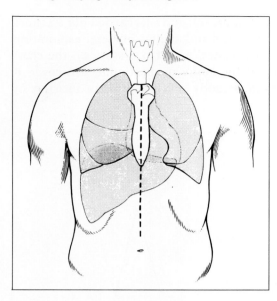

Fig. 2. Incision in median sternotomy with possibility of extension to median upper abdominal laparotomy. Alterations in both hemithoraces, the mediastinum and the upper abdomen can be verified and operated on synchronously.

median sternotomy to a median upper abdominal laparotomy, if necessary, in unclear abdominal processes in the upper abdomen (fig. 2). For example, it is thus possible in preoperatively unclear findings to arrive at a more precise appraisal of the upper abdominal organs (especially the liver but also the adrenals) than in a transdiaphragmatic laparotomy after lateral thoracotomy (fig. 3. a, b). Surgical operation such as atypical liver resections or (after appropriate mobilization) even anatomical segment resections of the liver can thus be carried out in conditions of good visibility. Retroperitoneal lymphadenectomy can be carried out at the same time as a mediastinal lymphadenectomy as well as intrapulmonary resection of metastases via a combined median thoracolaparotomy in metastases of testicular teratomas after semicastration, as recommended for the first time by Merrin and Takita [4].

In 15% of our patients, we also carried out laparotomy after median thoracotomy. In 4 cases, an atypical liver resection and in 2 cases a retroperitoneal lymphadenectomy was performed.

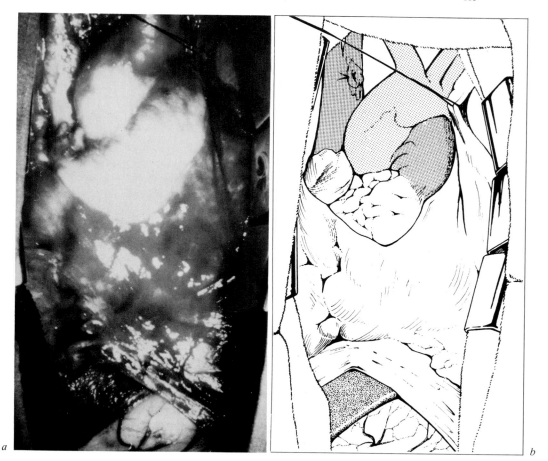

a   *b*

Fig. 3. a, b Site after median sternotomy and upper abdominal laparotomy. The anonymous vein is resected and mediastinal lymphadenectomy is carried out. The pericardium has already been opened to dissect the hilar structures. The left liver lobe and the stomach are visible.

Technical Aspects of Resection of Metastases via Median Thoracotomy

In surgery of metastases, artificial ventilation of adults and children should be performed on principle via a double-lumen tube (fig. 4) so that a unilateral ventilation can be administered. Alternatively, it is

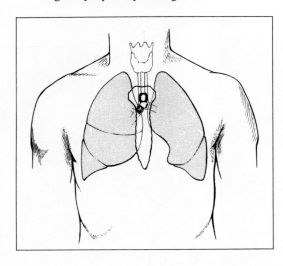

Fig. 4. Double-lumen tube for the unilateral ventilation of the lung which is always necessary in surgery of metastases.

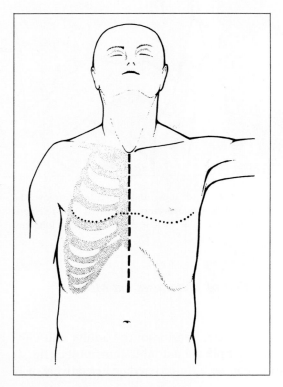

Fig. 5. Possibility of extension of median thoracotomy by an anterior thoracotomy in doorleaf manner.

possible to immobilize the lung with the technically more elaborate one-sided high-frequency jet ventilation.

In order to obtain an adequate approach to the lung roots and to the parenchyma from median, the thorax must be spread out wide. To this end, a sufficient prolongation of the incision into the median upper abdomen is necessary, and occasionally the fascia must also be divided. If laparotomy is not planned, the peritoneum should remain closed. The spreading of the halves of the sternum must be carried out slowly, since there is danger of tearing the anonymous vein and its opening into the superior vena cava if spreading is too fast. If the local conditions make this necessary, median thoracotomy can be extended in the form of doorleaves by an anterior thoracotomy (fig. 5). In such a case, attention must be paid not to damage the parasternal structures on both sides (fig. 6). After longitudinal division of the sternum, the retrosternally situated structures are exposed and the parietal pleura is dissected bluntly (fig. 7). For the further course of the operation, it has proved to be advantageous to expose the anonymous vein carefully in its course. Attention must be paid to the thymus vein opening caudally into the anonymous vein. Suspiciously enlarged lymph nodes of the anterior

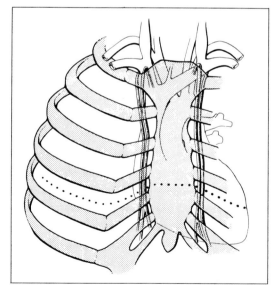

Fig. 6. Danger to the internal thoracic artery and veins passing parasternally on both sides in transverse sternotomy.

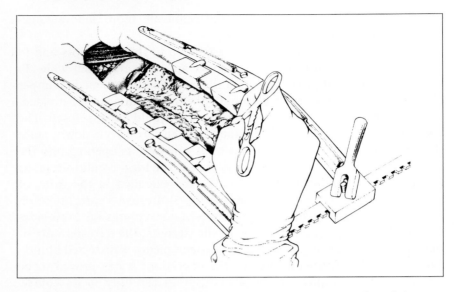

Fig. 7. Blunt dissection of the parietal pleura. The anonymous vein and the anterior mediastinal lymphatic trunk on top of it are shown.

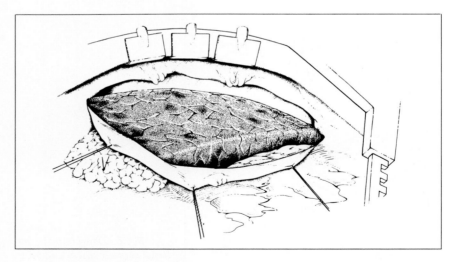

Fig. 8. The left pleural cavity is open. Pleurae, mediastinum, and lungs are inspected and palpated gently.

mediastinal lymphatic tract running along the anonymous vein are extirpated. If the operation site makes this necessary, the anonymous vein can be severed. In tumor processes infiltrating the parietal pleura, a primary extrapleural procedure must be carried out as in decortication. If the tumor process infiltrates the chest wall, circumscribed en-bloc resections of the chest wall including the corresponding parts of the ribs are also possible in the posterior thorax with a careful extrapleural procedure. In infiltrations of the chest wall over a larger area, it is possible that an extension of the thoracotomy in the form of doorleaves may become necessary.

To open the pleural cavity from the mediastinum, the mediastinal pleura should be severed in such a way that the pleural margin in the direction of the ribs and sternum remain sufficiently wide in order to enable good closure after completion of the operation. Cranially, care must be taken not to damage the phrenic nerve passing ventrally. If the pleural cavities are opened (fig. 8) the parietal pleura is initially investigated for tumor metastases. There is subsequent careful inspection of the mediastinal and hilar lymph nodes. Suspicious lymph nodes are extirpated. Afterwards, both lungs are inspected in accordance with the plan by two surgeons in sequence in the ventilated and atelectatic state. The severance of the pulmonary ligament can facilitate the access to the more distant regions of the lung in the lower lobe. The palpation must be carried out very carefully and if possible with little traumatization in order to avoid the development of interstitial edema with its negative effects on the postoperative phase.

This part of the operation is especially important in two respects. On the one hand, one must ensure that all the metastases present including those not diagnosed preoperatively are indeed identified, since otherwise the potentially curative approach to therapy is lost. On the other hand, the non-damaging palpation enables a reduction of the number of postoperative complications with persistent respiratory insufficiency. Suspect foci must be carefully marked. The side of the lung on which it is expected that less parenchyma will have to be removed is operated on first, so that in unilateral ventilation as much respiratory surface as possible is available on the contralateral side.

For this purpose, the lung must be mobilized first of all. After severance of the pulmonary ligament, the hilus is mobilized from the back with blunt finger dissection. For dissection on the parenchyma, the respective lung is luxated forward by the insertion of abdominal swabs

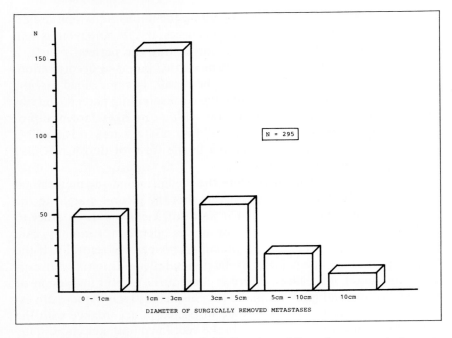

Fig. 9. Frequency distribution of the diameters of the pulmonary metastases removed. If several metastases were resected in one operation, the largest diameter in each case is specified.

into the dorsal pleural cavity. By a too severe luxation, especially on the left side, there may be kinking of the large pulmonary vessels, especially of the veins at the hilus as well as to the right of the vena cava. As a consequence of this, cardiac arrhythmias may occur. Arrhythmias may also occur in the intrapericardial and extrapericardial dissection on the pulmonary hilus. In our patients, bradycardias occurred in 17% of the cases, and there was a marked fall in blood pressure in addition in 7%.

These disorders can mostly be eliminated by reluxation of the lungs into the pleural cavities. The arrhythmias occur above all in forward luxation of the left lower lobe of the lung, and especially in cardiac enlargements, so that in these cases an extension of the thoracotomy in the form of doorleaves may become necessary transsternally to lateral between the fourth and fifth rib or the fifth and sixth rib in these cases (fig. 5). Since the majority of the metastases to be removed are smaller tumor metastases (fig. 9), these can be mostly removed by smaller resection techniques such as atypical and segment resections as well as enucleations (table III) which can be performed without effort on the lung luxated forward (fig. 10). So far, it could not be demonstrated that the anatomical segment or lobe resection is superior to radical atypical resection with regard to life expectancy in surgery of metastases both in the lungs and in the liver [6].

Differences in the survival rates depending on the resection technique were also not found in our own patients. Thus the small and moderately large metastases in the lung periphery at the front as well as at the back are removed via the usual clip resections or using the suture apparatus. Enucleations are sufficiently radical only in metastases of tough consistency with a distinct delimitation from the surrounding parenchyma, as is frequently the case in metastases of chondrosarcomas, for example. In deep enucleations and deep wedge resections as well as in anatomical resection, e.g. of the segment no. 6 with the technically sophisticated dissection from the front, above all on the left side, it is recommended that the pulmonary artery and the pulmonary vein be

Table III. Resection techniques in operations performed for pulmonary metastases. Where a combination of several techniques during one operation was used, the largest technique is specified

Resection techniques	All thoracotomies		Median thoracotomies		Lateral thoracotomies	
	n	%	n	%	n	%
Wedge, segment resection Enucleation	194	66	73	38	121	62
Lobectomy*	84	29	16	19	68	81
Bilobectomy*	10	3	3	30	7	70
Pneumonectomy*	3	1	–	–	3	100
Mediastinal lymph node Extirpation	4	1	–	–	4	100
Total	295	100	92	31	203	69

*including 28 (9.5%) broncho- and angioplastic operations

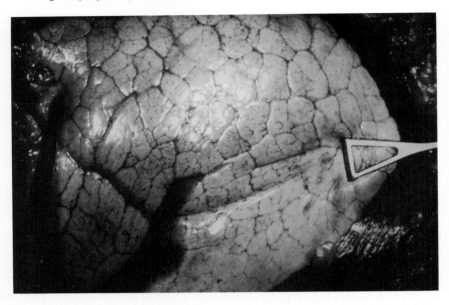

Fig. 10. The lung luxated forward into the anterior mediastinum. The two visible metastases can be readily removed via clamp resection.

clamped off after intrapericardial dissection. Injuries to the phrenic nerve must be avoided.

The operation can be performed in tissue practically 'empty of blood', since the blood stagnating within the lungs runs out after splitting of the parenchyma. Opened intersegmental veins and arterial branches can be dealt with precisely without damaging them and intraparenchymatous hemorrhages complicating the postoperative course can be avoided.

If a shunt volume which is too large occurs in unilateral ventilation, it is sometimes imperative to clamp off the pulmonary artery supplying the collapsed lungs when a dangerous oxygen undersaturation arises, since only in this way can the venous admixture be altered in such a way that a normal blood oxygenation with low FIO_2 values can be attained again (fig. 11).

In about one-third of the patients (table III), a lobectomy had to be carried out owing to the size, number or central position of the metastases. A bilobectomy or pneumonectomy was only performed in very

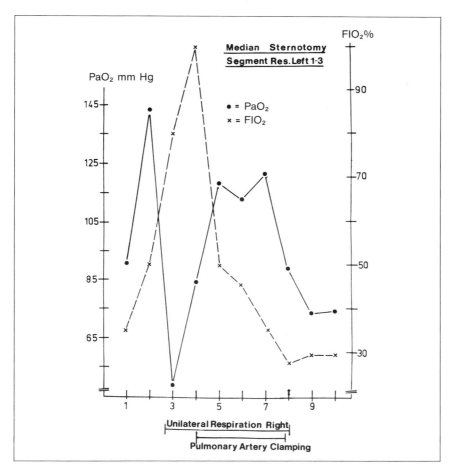

Fig. 11. Median sternotomy with resection of segments 1–3 on the left. On the ordinate on the left side, the arterial oxygen pressure values PaO$_2$, and on the right side the FIO$_2$ values are plotted. Below the abscissa, the beginning of the unilateral ventilation of the right lung and the ligation of the pulmonary artery are marked. After onset of unilateral ventilation of the right lung, the arterial oxygen pressure falls from 90 mm Hg to 49 mm Hg despite high inspiratory oxygen percentages. The ligation of the pulmonary artery of the collapsed side brings about an immediate rise of the values of arterial oxygen pressure owing to elimination of the shunt, so that the inspiratory oxygen concentration can be reduced to 30% with maintenance of normal values of arterial oxygen pressure despite unilateral ventilation.

rare cases. In view of a possible operation on recurrences and possibly postoperative chemotherapy, pneumonectomy should be obviated if possible by a bronchoplastic or angioplastic procedure, which we were able to perform in 9% of the median thoracotomies. For such larger resections, the mediastinum must be exposed and a clear view of the central structures must be aimed for.

Whereas on the right the dissection of the hilus structures as well as closure of the bronchus from the front are not more problematical than from the lateral thoracotomy, the conditions are more difficult on the left side owing to the forward luxation of the heart.

First of all, the mediastinal pleura must be exposed (fig. 12). To dissect the left root of the lung, the phrenic nerve and vagus nerve must be exposed so as not to damage them. The lymph nodes accompanying the phrenic nerve may be infiltrated with metastases and must be extirpated when this is suspected. In isolation of the lymph nodes by dissection, the vessels accompanying the nerve may be injured, which leads to an at least transient disorder of function. For preparation of the lung root, it is to be recommended that a broad longitudinal incision is made in the anterior mediastinal pleura below the phrenic nerve after posterior mobilization. Afterwards, the pericardium is split wide open, attention being paid once more to the phrenic nerve and the recurrent nerve. It has proved to be advantageous to carry out this dissection from cranial to caudal, so that the second assistant stands on the right beside the surgeon. The hilar structures are largely dissected bluntly from intrapericardial. After adequate mobilization of the ascending aorta and afterwards of the pulmonary trunk, dissection of the pulmonary artery on the left side is carried out from the upper pulmonary vein (fig. 13). For further dissection, the lung is replaced into the pleural cavity. The traction on the hilus which this causes leads to tension in the vessels, so

---

Fig. 12. Dissection of the left mediastinal pleura (with abundant attached fat tissue) in the direction of the left hilus. The phrenic nerve with accompanying lymph nodes and the vagus nerve situated farther dorsally are shown.

Fig. 13. After the pericardium has been opened wide, the left upper hilus pole is shown. The pulmonary artery including the origin of the upper lobe segment artery 1–3 and upper lobe vein are dissected. Ligament of Botalli and vagus nerve with recurrent laryngeal nerve are visible.

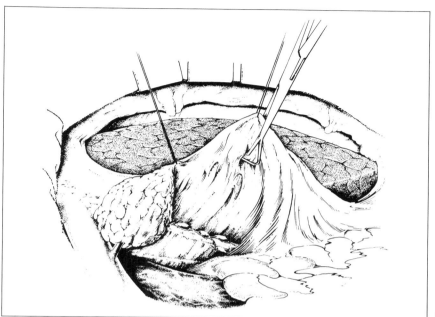

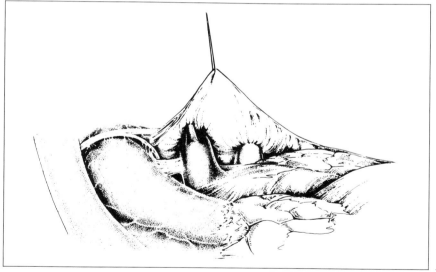

that they can be visualized more easily and more clearly. The pulmonary artery is dissected at the upper hilus pole towards the periphery as far as possible to the back at the bottom (fig. 14. a, b). For example, in a planned resection of the lower lobes, the lower part of the pulmonary artery is visualized from the lobe fissure. The branches of the pulmonary artery then also indicate the course of the lobe bronchus as well as of the bronchus of the 6th segment. For upper lobe resection, the upper bronchus can be readily exposed by division of the upper lobe vein. Anatomical segment resections can also be carried out readily after dissection of the pulmonary artery (fig. 15. a, b). After the end of the operation, the pericardium must be carefully closed again leaving behind a small window with a view to a possible resternotomy. In principle, resternotomies can be carried out without major problems in recurrences, which has also been confirmed by other authors [3, 5] in large patient series. However, the operation is easier when the pericardium was not opened in the previous operation [3].

So far, systematic mediastinal lymphadenectomy is not a fundamental component of operations on pulmonary metastases. We found lymph node metastases in 20% of the potentially curative resections. The underlying primary tumors were mainly testicular teratomas, hypernephromas and colorectal carcinomas. These are tumors in all of which a purely lymphogenic metastatic spreading into the lungs is possible as an alternative to the probably more frequent hematogenic route. Especially after removal of pulmonary metastases of these primary tumors, the mediastinum should hence be dissected with a subsequent systematic lymphadenectomy. The bilateral paratracheal and tracheobronchial region can be exposed more readily with an anterior approach than via lateral thoracotomy (fig. 16). For dissection of the bifurcation and the infrabifurcal region, the pericardium must be slit open wide at the front and the back, and the trunk of the right pulmonary artery must be mobilized intrapericardially. The left paratracheal and tracheobronchial lymph nodes are located and extirpated either from the right between the aorta and the superior vena cava in the same way as the right paratracheal and tracheobronchial lymph nodes, or are to be reached above all in the region of the bifurcation on the left between the aortic arch and the main trunk of the pulmonary artery medial to the ligament of Botalli (fig. 17). On the right side, the corresponding lymph nodes are to be found medial to the superior vena cava above and below the anonymous vein (fig. 18. a, b).

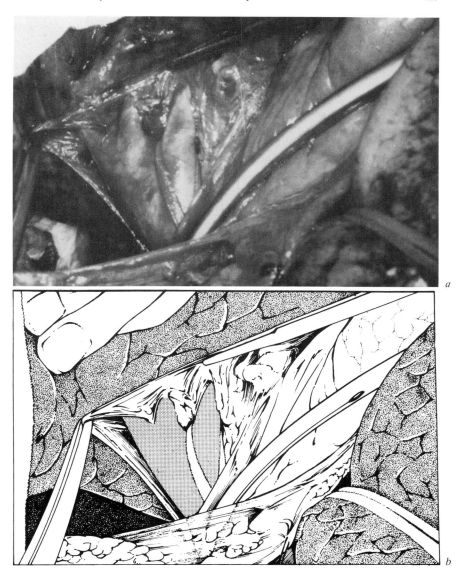

Fig. 14. a, b In the lung luxated back into the pleural cavity, the pulmonary artery is dissected far to dorsal. The objective is a 2-segment resection in order to remove the large solitary metastases of a colorectal carcinoma. The pulmonary arterial trunk is ligated, segmental artery 1–3 is snared, and the segment artery 2 and lower lobe artery are visible.

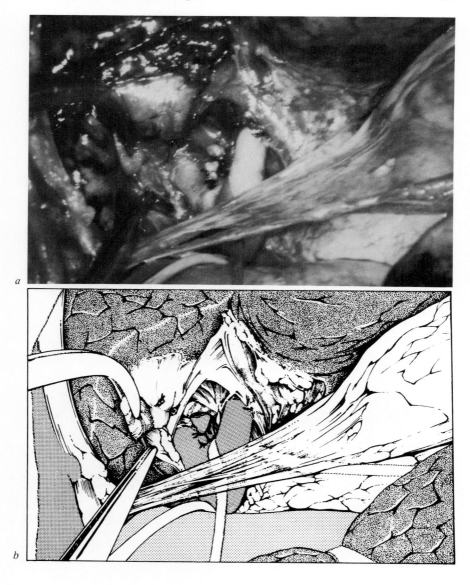

Fig. 15. a, b Site after resection of the segment no. 2 on the left. The segmental artery 1–3 is snared and the lower lobe artery is visible. The upper lobe bronchus is visible under the ligated segment artery 2.

The removal of lymph node metastases present paraesophagally from the deep mediastinum in the section below the bifurcation can be very difficult. In such cases, it is recommended that the lower right mediastinum be dissected from below, to which end an anterolateral doorleaf thoracotomy may be necessary.

Conclusion

The duration of postoperative ventilation is very much longer after operations of metastases via median thoracotomy [3] than after lateral thoracotomy (table IV). The median thoracotomy with simultaneous bilateral exploration or operation of the lungs and the mediastinum entails a more substantial surgical trauma than lateral thoracotomy with unilateral operation. This also becomes visible in the markedly raised 30-day lethality of 5.4% as compared to 2.4% in lateral thoracotomy

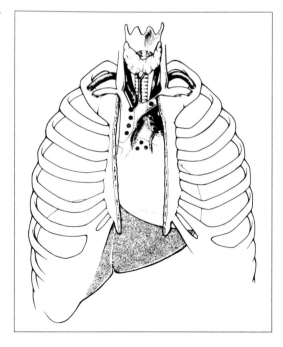

Fig. 16. Topographical correlations of the aorta with supra-aortic branches, superior vena cava with tributaries and the trachea with bifurcation and main bronchi (dashed lines) situated deep in the mediastinum behind the large vessels. The circles mark the topographical position of the lymph nodes paratracheally and tracheobronchially on both sides as well as below the bifurcation.

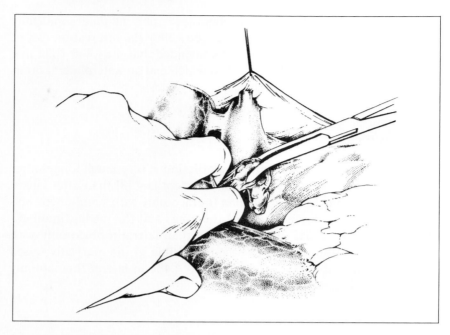

Fig. 17. Paratracheal and tracheobronchial lymphadenectomy on the left side. The left hand of the surgeon draws the aortic arch upwards.

(table V). The surgical risk of operations of metastases is accordingly about twice as high after median thoracotomy than after lateral thoracotomy and unilateral operation. Here, a more refined technique with improvement of results can be expected in the future owing to increasing experience. With regard to the individual resection techniques, an

Fig. 18. a, b Localization of the paratracheal and tracheobronchial lymph nodes on the right side. View from the head of the patient. In the triangle between aortic arch, anonymous vein and superior vena cava, the trachea with bifurcation and branching point of the upper lobe bronchus is situated deep on the right. Perpendicularly in front of it rises the azygos vein. If the superior vena cava is drawn away to dextrolateral for paratracheal and tracheobronchial lymphadenectomy on the right side, a tear of the azygos vein rising perpendicularly from the depths in front of the right upper lobe bronchus can easily result.

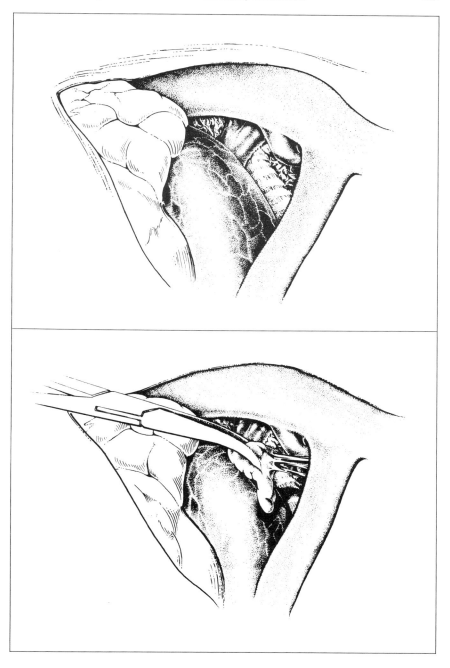

Table IV. Postoperative ventilation period following operations on pulmonary metastases

Postop. respiratory therapy	Median thoracotomy (n = 92)		Lateral thoracotomy (n = 212)	
	n	%	n	%
None	5	5.4	157	74.1
Up to 12 hours	50	54.3	47	22.2
Up to 24 hours	30	32.6	6	2.8
Up to 5 days	2	2.2	2	1.0
> 5 days	5	5.4	–	–

Table V. 30-day lethality of operations on pulmonary metastases classified according to resection techniques and approach

	n	%
Resection techniques (n = 304)		
Wedge, segment resection, enucleation	3	1.5
Lobectomy	4	4.8
Bilobectomy	2	20.0
Pneumonectomy	1	33.0
Approach (n = 304)		
Lateral thoracotomy	5	2.4
Median thoracotomy	5	5.4
Total	10	3.3

Table VI. Advantages of median thoracotomy as compared to lateral thoracotomy

1. Simultaneous establishment of findings in both hemithoraces and the mediastinum
2. Possibility of extension to median abdominal laparotomy
3. Avoidance of a secondarily inoperable situation
4. Low subjective stress of the patient (pain, psychological)

above-average high perioperative lethality was found for bilobectomy and pneumonectomy (20% and 30% respectively). However, in view of the small number of 10 and 3 patients respectively, these results are not of general validity. Overall, the 30-day lethality resection of pulmonary metastases is 3.3% in our patients. To summarize, in view of the advantages specified (table VI) at present, we hence regard median thoracotomy as the most suitable approach in operations on metastases in the lungs and mediastinum.

References

1   Chang, A. E.; Schaner, E. G.; Concle, D. M.: Evaluation of computed tomography in the detection of pulmonary metastases. Cancer 43: 913–916 (1979).

2   Friedmann, G.; Bohndorf, K.; Krüger, J.: Radiology of pulmonary metastases: comparison of imaging techniques with operative findings. J. thorac. cardiovasc. Surg. 34: 120–124 (1986).

3   Johnston, M. R.: Median sternotomy for resection of pulmonary metastases. J. thorac. cardiovasc. Surg. 85: 516–522 (1983).

4   Merrin, C.; Takita, H.; Beckley, S.; Kassis, J.: Treatment of recurrent and widespread testicular tumor by radical reductive surgery and multiple sequential chemotherapy. J. Urol. 117: 291–295 (1977).

5   Regal, A. M.; Hart, T.; Takita, H.: Median sternotomy for resection of metastatic lung lesions Abstracts, XIV. World Congress on Diseases of the Chest, Toronto (1982).

6   Schildberg, F. W.; Meyer, G.; Wenk, H.: Der Stellenwert der Chirurgie bei der Therapie von Tumormetastasen; in Eigler, Peiper, Schildberg et al., Stand und Gegenstand der chirurgischen Forschung, pp. 457–487. (Springer, Berlin, Heidelberg, New York, Tokyo 1986).

7   Takita, H.; Merrin, C.; Didolkar, M. S. et al.: The surgical management of multiple lung metastases. Ann. thor. Surg. 24: 359–363 (1977).

8   Vogt-Moykopf, I.; Meyer, G.; Merkle, N. M. et al.: Late results of surgical treatment of pulmonary metastases. J. thorac. cardiovasc. Surg. 34: 143–148 (1986).

Prof. Dr. I. Vogt-Moykopf, Chirurgische Abteilung, Thoraxklinik der LVA Baden, Krankenhaus Rohrbach, Amalienstraße 5, D-6900 Heidelberg (FRG)

Contr. Oncol., vol. 30, pp. 132–137 (Karger, Basel 1988)

Radiotherapy of Lung Metastases

H. Sack, W. Alberti

University Clinic for Radiotherapy, Essen, FRG

Lung metastases are part of a generalized malignant disease. Radiotherapy, being a mainly local treatment modality, is therefore only sometimes indicated and today is not in competition with the operative removal of lung metastases as it was in the past. In contrast to the situation 10–20 years ago, surgery of solitary lung metastases has developed into a routine treatment modality which offers the patient a curative step with low morbidity and mortality. In multiple lung metastases chemotherapy has become an effective weapon, so that radiotherapy often remains in the background. Approximately one in three tumor patients has to expect lung metastases in the course of his disease. From the radiotherapeutic point of view, the number of publications on this subject is small and reflects the minor importance of radiation therapy.

Treatment of Solitary Lung Metastases by Radiotherapy Alone

Radiotherapy is not in competition with the surgical removal of solitary metastases. Indications for radiation treatment are
- solitary metastases when surgery is not possible for functional or other reasons,
- metastases not responding to chemo- or hormonal therapy,
- metastases which are not considered to be effectively treated by chemotherapy, for example in malignant melanoma or in renal carcinoma, and
- when chemotherapy has no indication.

Radiotherapy of solitary lung metastases is effective. A dose of 50 Gy in 17 fractions over 3 weeks or 60 Gy in 20 fractions over 4 weeks is given depending on the size of the metastases. The local recurrence rate is less than 5%. However, the target volume has to be chosen generously in order to include the whole tumor and to be sure that the metastasis remains in the target volume in spite of the respiratory movements of the lung. The sequel to the radiation treatment is always a circumscribed lung fibrosis which is adapted to the size of the treatment volume. It becomes visible on an X-ray film about 3 months later.

Again and again patients who suffer from a metastasizing tumor which is controlled by chemotherapy outside the lung but is not controlled or even growing in the lung are referred to radiotherapy. In this case it is important to differentiate between whether the persisting lung metastasis consists of active tumor tissue and whether the malignant cells have disappeared after successful chemotherapy although remaining benign cells continue to appear as tumor. We often make this observation in lung metastases of malignant teratoma. But there are without doubt lung metastases which do not respond to chemotherapy, in contrast to metastases outside the lung, because they consist of less sensitive cell clones. These metastases can be irradiated successfully. On the other hand, an operative removal of these metastases may not be a good recommendation to the patient with a known generalized tumor and an uncertain prognosis.

In the case of generalized metastases, radiation therapy of a few lung metastases may be advisable, especially in the hilar region when chemotherapy is not considered to be successful. This is generally the case in malignant melanoma and also in other tumors. Here radiotherapy has a palliative character and is intended to prevent discomfort by growing metastases. The same holds true for patients in whom chemotherapy is contraindicated. An example may demonstrate this: A patient was suffering from a metastasizing breast carcinoma with two solitary lung metastases. For other reasons she had a persistent ulcus cruris which was aggravated during chemotherapy, forcing a stop to chemotherapy, whereupon we irradiated these lung metastases, although it is quite clear that new metastases outside the irradiated area will appear in a short time. The patient had a small chance of having solitary metastases, so we took advantage of this opportunity by applying radiation treatment which did not involve much inconvenience.

In our opinion, the criteria for the selection of patients with solitary lung metastases for radiotherapy are: when lung metastases are detected before or together with the primary tumor, or when the latent period between the treatment of the primary tumor and the manifestation of lung metastases is only a few months. Under these conditions it is most probable that other metastases will appear soon, so an operative removal is not advisable.

Treatment of Multiple Lung Metastases with Radiotherapy Alone

Radiotherapy alone cannot control a generalized tumor which is only detectable in the lung. The reason is that other occult metastases remain without treatment and that the tolerance of the normal lung tissue against radiation is limited. The literature overview given in table I lists papers from the early 1970s when chemotherapy was not as efficient as it is nowadays. However, table I also demonstrates that 2 of 7 patients with Ewing's sarcoma and some others with different tumors survived 2 years without evidence of disease. According to our own experience, too, radiotherapy is occasionally successful, but as a rule it is only able to make limited improvements on the survival rate. The failures can be attributed to metastases in other organs or recurrences in the lung. When irradiating the whole lung the radiation tolerance of the

Table I. Survival of patients with lung metastases after radiotherapy alone (historical data)

Author	Year	Tumor	Patients (n)	2-year survival (%)	Lethal pneumonitis
Margolis and Phillips	1973	Ewing's	7	29	0
Wara et al.	1974	Wilms'	5	0	0
Newton	1973	sarcoma	6	0	0
		testicle	11	27	0
		Ewing's	7	15	0
		Hodgkin's	2	100	0
Hussey et al.	1971	Wilms'	1	0	0
Monson et al.	1972	Wilms'	89	11	./.

normal lung tissue is limited, and above a dose of 17.5 Gy the rate of lung fibrosis increases rapidly. By contrast, smaller portals allow higher doses, as are used in solitary metastases, for which the control rate is higher.

Adjuvant Radiotherapy

The failures in the local treatment of osteogenic sarcomas are based on the late appearance of lung metastases. Before the era of chemotherapy, 60–80% of the patients died because of lung metastases not detectable at primary treatment. Two controlled studies were started to find out if radiotherapy of the whole lung during primary treatment – when lung metastases are not apparent – can reduce the rate of lung metastases developing later. In the EORTC study 20 Gy in 2 weeks were applied to the whole lung, whereby the rate of lung metastases which developed later was reduced to half of that in the control group. Similar results were shown by Newton and Spittle [7] when they applied 19.5 Gy in 13 fractions with 1.5 Gy as single dose. Today an efficient chemotherapy is available, which itself causes toxic side-effects on the lungs and heart and therefore cannot continue to be used after radiotherapy failures; otherwise, high rates of complications can be expected. Thus, we do not use primary irradiation of the lung as an adjuvant therapy for these reasons.

Combined Radio- and Chemotherapy

Table II gives an overview of the amelioration of the 2-year survival rate when combining radio- and chemotherapy in the treatment of lung metastases. The better results can probably be attributed to the treatment (by chemotherapy) of foci outside the irradiated volume and of remaining cells within the irradiated volume which have not been lethally damaged. The best results are shown in tumors which preferably or exclusively metastasize into the lung. In Wilms' tumor, radiotherapy of the whole lung is a well-established treatment modality in many centers. The whole lung is irradiated in patients with Wilms' tumor, independent of the number and distribution of lung metastases, in order to be sure to include all not visible microscopically small metastases in the target

Table II. Survival of patients with lung metastases of Wilms' tumor after combined chemo- and radiotherapy

Author	Year	Patients (n)	2-year survival (%)	Lethal pneumonitis
Wara et al.	1974	13	62	1
Cassady et al.	1973	42	48	4
Monson et al.	1972	168	42	./.
Baeza et al.	1975	9	45	3

volume. Daily doses of 1.0−1.5 Gy are applied. In children, the total dose should not exceed 12 Gy; otherwise, signs of pneumonitis will be observed in more than 10% of the patients.

The example of a 27-month-old boy suffering from Wilms' tumor with bilateral lung metastases will demonstrate the problems of this treatment modality. The boy was treated with cyclophosphamide, actinomycin D, vincristine, and adriamycin, and a partial remission was achieved. Because lung metastases still existed, we irradiated the left lung with a total dose of 12 Gy in 12 fractions of 1 Gy. Additionally, we irradiated a large metastasis with 20 Gy over a small field. The boy survived 26 months and died of an interstitial pneumonia. The combination of radio- and chemotherapy in the treatment of the whole lung continues to be a problem and can only be recommended in studies or in single cases as a palliative treatment.

On the whole, radiation therapy only plays a small role in the treatment of lung metastases. Data in the literature on radiation treatment of lung metastases, on combined modalities, and on adjuvant irradiation are of more historical than current value.

References

1   Baeza, M. R.; Barkley, H. T.; Fernandez, C. H.: Total lung irradiation in the treatment of pulmonary metastases. Radiology 116: 151−154 (1975).
2   Cassady, J. R.; Tefft, M.; Filler, R. M. et al.: Considerations in the radiation therapy of Wilms' tumor. Cancer 32: 598−608 (1973).
3   Hussey, D. H.; Castro, J. R.; Sullivan, M. P.; Sutow, W. W.: Radiation therapy in management of Wilms' tumor. Radiology 101: 663−668 (1971).

4   Margolis, L. W.; Phillips, T. L.: Whole-lung irradiation for metastatic tumor. Radiology *93:* 1173−1179 (1969).
5   Monson, K. J.; Brand, W. N.; Boggs, J. D.: Results of small-field irradiation of apparent solitary metastases from Wilms' tumor. Radiology *104:* 157−160 (1972).
6   Newton, K. A.: The Colston Papers No. 24; in Price, Ross, Bone, p. 307 (Butterworth, London 1973).
7   Newton, K. A.; Spittle, M. F.: An analysis of 40 cases treated by total thoracic irradiation. Clin. Radiol. *20:* 19−22 (1969).
8   Wara, W. M.; Margolis, L. W.; Smith, W. B. et al.: Treatment of metastatic Wilms' tumor. Radiology *112:* 695−697 (1974).

Professor Dr. Horst Sack, Strahlenklinik des Universitätsklinikums, Hufelandstr. 55, D-4300 Essen 1 (FRG)

Contr. Oncol., vol. 30, pp. 138–142 (Karger, Basel 1988)

Therapy of Patients with Lung Metastases – the Internist's Point of View

D. K. Hossfeld

Department of Oncology and Hematology, Medical Clinic, University of Hamburg, FRG

This is not an easy subject to deal with, since *the* therapy for patients with lung metastases does not exist. On the other hand, this topic represents a rather frequent problem; in the author's experience, about 15% of the patients who seek the advice of a medical oncologist do so because of lung metastases.

A quite large number of questions must be raised before appropriate therapy can be considered for the individual patient with lung metastases, among which the following are of particular importance:

– Is the primary tumor known?

– Could the lung deposits be related to a non-malignant process or to a hitherto unknown secondary neoplasia?

– What is the histology, grading, tumor-marker status of the primary tumor?

– What is the date of diagnosis of the primary tumor and the duration of the metastasis-free interval?

– What is the extent of lung metastases (number and size)?

– How are the dynamics of metastases – do they increase fast, slowly, or not at all; do they even regress spontaneously?

– Are the metastases limited to the lungs?

– What type of treatment was given for the primary tumor – was it with or without adjuvant chemotherapy?

The therapeutic strategy finally chosen must be a synthesis of the answers to such questions. Obviously, what is needed is not only considerable personal experience but also the consultation of other medical faculties.

In this contribution, the author anticipates that the tumor responsible for the lung metastases is known from the patient's previous history. Yet it should be briefly indicated that the possibility that the lung deposits may be due to a non-malignant process or to a secondary tumor must always be kept in mind. Particularly patients with carcinomas of the oropharynx, mammary glands, ovaries, colon and endometrium uteri run a high risk of developing secondary cancers [1]. It goes without saying that it does have therapeutic and prognostic consequences knowing whether the lung metastases are derived from a known mammary cancer or a so far unknown colon cancer. A case in point would be the following: During the following 10 years after the diagnosis of breast cancer, a 62-year-old woman was diagnosed as having three additional cancers, namely cancer of the colon ascendens, cancer of the sigma and cancer of the endometrium uteri. A routine chest X-ray disclosed multiple lung metastases. In this situation CEA and histology could not contribute to the question as to the origin of the metastases. The estrogen receptor status was determined by means of immunohistochemistry on a small tissue sample obtained by percutaneous fine-needle aspiration. The test was positive. The lung metastases were thought to be derived from breast cancer; Tamoxifen was given, and a long-lasting remission could be achieved. A 72-year-old man with kidney cancer may serve as another example: He complained about back pain. A bone scan showed multiple hot spots. A greatly elevated acid phosphatase level led to the diagnosis of prostatic cancer, and the patient was treated successfully with hormone therapy.

The knowledge of the exact histology of the primary tumor, its grading and other tumor characteristics influence the therapeutic decision, particularly in sarcomas and germ cell tumors, less so in epithelial tumors. In patients with yolk-sac tumors surgery has priority, while in patients with embryonic carcinoma chemotherapy should be given initially. If the receptor status of the breast cancer was positive, ablative or additive hormone therapy would be the initial treatment of choice provided that other prognostic factors would not speak against it.

Even if there are no doubts about the relationship between the lung metastases and the known primary tumor, it is not always successful to assume that the metastases mirror the characteristics of the primary tumor. The heterogeneity of tumors must be taken into consideration, from which follows that the metastases may be more or less differentiated than the primary tumor, that they can be tumor-marker negative

or positive, etc. Recently, one of our patients with osteosarcoma underwent thoracotomy because a single nodule had appeared in his right upper lung one year after he had been taken off adjuvant chemotherapy.
Histology revealed a fibrous histiocytoma. A review of slides of the
primary tumor confirmed osteosarcoma with fibrous histiocytoma in
one tiny, minute area.

The interval between the diagnosis of the primary disease and the
appearance of metastatic disease is of clinical and prognostic importance, although the author is aware of the contradicting opinions with
regard to this topic [2, 3]. Cum granu salis it can be said that a short
interval not only points to the metastatic nature of lung nodules and
their relationship to the previously diagnosed cancer, but also to the necessity of giving systemic therapy as initial treatment. A long interval
makes it necessary to take into consideration secondary cancers and
benign lung disease, and in such a situation thoracotomy is of considerable value, as it serves diagnostic as well as (in some instances, definite)
therapeutic purposes.

Before one or the other therapeutic decision is made, it is advisable
to gain an impression about the growth potential of the metastases by
repeating X-rays or CT scan at appropriate intervals. At the same time,
the question of whether the metastatic process is limited to the lungs or
has spread to other organs as well has to be addressed. If the lung
metastases have clearly progressed within an observation period of 4−8
weeks and if the disease has been detected also in other organs, then systemic therapeutic measures will have to be preferred over local (surgery,
radiation) ones. In case the lung metastases are stationary, a 'wait-and-
see policy' can be the best treatment. This type of treatment is probably
the most difficult one of all, since it requires that both the physician and
the patient accept the limitations of present-day medicine. However, in
some very rare cases such a policy may be very rewarding when a partial
or even complete spontaneous regression of the metastases can be observed! Every experienced oncologist has made such observations, but
hardly anyone dares to publish such cases for fear of being considered
a storyteller since it is not possible to offer a scientifically based expla-
nation for it. Spontaneous regression of lung metastases has been noted
most frequently in patients with kidney cancer, followed by patients
with melanoma and testicular cancer [4]. In patients with testicular cancer it is certainly not advisable to wait for this very rare event of spontaneous regression, since very effective chemotherapy is available nowa-

days. This situation is certainly not true for kidney cancer and melanoma, and it may be added parenthetically that a remarkable parallelism appears to exist between tumors with a tendency towards spontaneous regression and those which respond somewhat to biological response modifiers. The author has seen 3 patients with spontaneous regression of metastases during the last 8 years. The first patient, a 25-year-old woman, had surgery and irradiation for treatment of an anaplastic carcinoma of the oropharynx. Multiple lung metastases appeared 6 months later which increased in number and size during the following 3 months. Within the next 12 months they disappeared completely. The second patient had multiple lung and liver metastases at the time of surgery due to a bleeding kidney cancer. He received 2 courses of vinblastin by continuous infusion and went into a complete pulmonary remission. Since none of the 20 patients subsequently treated with this regimen had responded, we are inclined to believe that this patient, too, had a spontaneous remission. The third patient had undergone emergency surgery because of an acute abdomenal condition. A perforated stomach ulcer and multiple liver metastases were found. The ulcer was excised and biopsies of liver metastases were taken. Histology revealed immunoblastic lymphoma of the stomach and the liver. Postoperative staging confirmed the liver lesions but no additional manifestations. Chemotherapy was planned. However, because the stomach ulcer persisted, it was decided to perform a gastrectomy first. At this time, 4 weeks after emergency laparotomy, the liver was free of disease macro- and microscopically. Chemotherapy was withheld. The patient continues to be in complete remission up to now (4 years after diagnosis).

The dynamic and the type of the disease as well as the patient's general condition should determine the therapeutic strategy to a much greater extent than the number and size of the lung metastases. Neither are multiple lung metastases as such a priori a clear-cut indication for chemotherapy, nor is a solitary lung metastasis an unambiguous indication for surgery. A patient who develops a single-lung metastasis a few months after the diagnosis of testicular cancer, stage I, and in whom the tumor markers rise again should undergo chemotherapy and not thoracotomy. A patient with late-appearing, multiple lung metastases following kidney cancer is a candidate for surgery. The difference between these two examples is the exquisite chemotherapy sensitivity of testicular cancer and the notorious resistance of kidney cancer to chemotherapy.

However, it must be kept in mind that in patients with lung metastases surgery and chemotherapy are not mutually exclusive. In patients with osteosarcoma, testicular cancer and certain soft-tissue sarcomas the strategy of initial chemotherapy and subsequent surgery has been shown to be particularly rewarding. However, to be curative this approach requires chemotherapy to be very effective. The hope to be curative by means of surgery after chemotherapy has failed, is unrealistic. We have lost all our patients with testicular cancer who had had surgery at a time when the tumor markers were still, even minimally, positive.

The author is convinced that in patients with malignant lymphoma involving intrathoracic organs surgery has only a diagnostic role to play. He believes that this is a domain of medical oncology. Whether indeed the prognosis of such patients has been improved by debulking surgery, as has been claimed by some surgeons, remains to be demonstrated conclusively. All these patients, even after extensive surgery, need chemo- and/or radiotherapy, and here again it is unknown that the effect of chemo-/radiotherapy can be improved by previous surgery.

The author's attitude toward surgical removal of lung metastases in patients with breast cancer is similarly skeptical. The few patients he knows all had recurrent disease after a short interval either in the lungs or in other organs, underscoring the experience that breast cancer, once metastasized, is a systemic disease. Thus, breast cancer patients with lung metastases should be subjected to systemic therapy. If they have had adjuvant chemotherapy, the selections of one or the other chemotherapy regimen may pose a problem. As a rule of thumb, it can be suggested that an alternative regimen should be used if the disease-free interval was short, while the original regimen can be reinstituted after a long interval.

References

1 Stoll, B. A. (ed.): Risk factors and multiple cancer (John Wiley, Chichester 1984).
2 Pilch, Y. H. (ed.): Surgical oncology (McGraw-Hill, New York 1984).
3 Roth, J. A.: Treatment of metastatic cancer to the lung; in DeVita, Hellmann, Rosenberd, Cancer. Principles and practice of oncology, pp. 2104–2117 (Lippincott, Philadelphia 1985).
4 Stoll, B. A. (ed.): Prolonged arrest of cancer (John Wiley, Chichester 1982).

Prof. Dr. med. D. K. Hossfeld, Abt. Onkologie und Hämatologie,
Medizinische Univ.-Klinik, Martinistr. 52, D-2000 Hamburg 20 (FRG)

Contr. Oncol., vol. 30, pp. 143–149 (Karger, Basel 1988)

Prognosis after Metastasis in Osteosarcoma: Experience from the COSS Studies[1]

G. Beron[a], K. Winkler[a], J. Beck[b], F. Berthold[c], W. Brandeis[d], V. Gerein[e], W. Havers[f], G. Henze[g], H. Jürgens[h], R. Kotz[i], G. Prindull[k], J. Ritter[l], L. Stengel-Rutkowski[m], J. Treuner[n], C. Urban[o], P. Weinel[p]

[a] Abteilung für pädiatrische Hämatologie und Onkologie, Universitäts-Kinderklinik, Hamburg, FRG, and
Universitäts-Kinderklinik
[b] Erlangen, [c] Gießen, [d] Heidelberg, [e] Frankfurt/M., [f] Essen, [g] Berlin,
[h] Düsseldorf, FRG
[i] Orthopädische Universitätsklinik Wien, Austria, and
Universitäts-Kinderklinik
[k] Göttingen, [l] Münster, [m] München, [n] Tübingen, FRG, [o] Graz, Austria,
[p] Hannover, FRG

Since the introduction of aggressive surgical removal of pulmonary metastases from osteosarcoma [1], the prognosis of the affected patients has improved dramatically. Long-term survival rates reported in several recently published single-institution series have been in the order of 30–40% [2]. Completeness of resection has been repeatedly demonstrated to be of the utmost prognostic importance, while the influence of other factors such as tumor doubling time, disease-free interval, multiplicity or bilaterality of lesions, and, last but not least, the exact contribution of chemotherapy to survival, remain controversial [3–6].

The following report summarizes our experience with the management of pulmonary metastases of osteosarcoma within the multi-institutional framework of the German/Austrian Cooperative Osteosarcoma Study (COSS) group.

[1] Presented in part at the Symposium 'Die Therapie von Lungenmetastasen im interdisziplinären Konzept', Heidelberg, June 1986.

Patients and Methods

We reviewed the data on clinical features, treatment and outcome of 54 unselected patients with osteogenic sarcoma metastatic to the lung who were enrolled in the prospective multicenter trials COSS-77 and COSS-80 between 1977 and 1982. These protocols as well as results in patients without evidence of metastases at the start of therapy have been published in detail previously [7, 8]. Of the 54 patients with pulmonary metastases, 7 were initially treated according to COSS-77 and the other 47 according to COSS-80. Thirty patients were male and 24 female. The median age was 14 years (range 5–55 years). Primary tumor sites were proximal femur (4 patients), distal femur (27), proximal tibia (6), distal and mid tibia (2 cases each), proximal fibula (1), proximal humerus (7), distal radius (2), clavicula (1), and pelvis (2 cases).

Synchronous primary tumor and pulmonary metastases were present in 16 patients. Eight patients had developed pulmonary metastases within 1–6 months after the diagnosis of the primary tumor, 18 within 7–12 months, 7 within 13–18 months, 2 within 19–24 months, and only 1 each after 30, 52, and 54 months. We reported on this group of patients previously [9], and the results are now updated as of October 1985.

Results

Table I gives a summary of the results. Four cases had to be excluded because of incomplete documentation of therapy and outcome.

Table I. Pulmonary metastases from osteosarcoma – summary of subgroups and treatment outcome

16 Synchronous 38 Metachronous	> 54 patients	
	4 not evaluable	
	21 no thoracotomy	1 NED
8 Synchronous 16 Metachronous	> 29 thoracotomy(-ies)	9 NED
	7 incomplete	1 NED
6 Synchronous 16 Metachronous	> 22 complete	8 NED
	9 solitary	3 NED
	4 with 2–5 nodules	2 NED
	9 with > 5 nodules	3 NED

NED = no evidence of disease

Twenty-one patients did not undergo thoracotomy, mostly because of far-advanced disease. Twenty of them have died, 19 from disease and 1 from a fatal methotrexate toxicity, while the only surviving patient had no evidence of disease 54 months after amputation for a distal femur lesion. He had undergone 8 months of chemotherapy (COSS-80, BCD arm), during which his synchronous multiple bilateral pulmonary nodules regressed completely.

Details of the surgical procedures in the remaining 29 cases were published earlier [9]. A total of 45 operations were performed, namely, 27 unilateral thoracotomies, 9 staged bilateral thoracotomies, 5 simultaneous bilateral thoracotomies, and 4 median sternotomies. Over 235 pulmonary nodules were resected (the exact number was not given in 2 patients with multiple lesions). Seven patients had a second and 3 patients a third, fourth, and fifth exploration respectively. Of these 29 patients, 9 survived with no evidence of disease, for an actuarial postmetastatic 5-year survival rate of 31%.

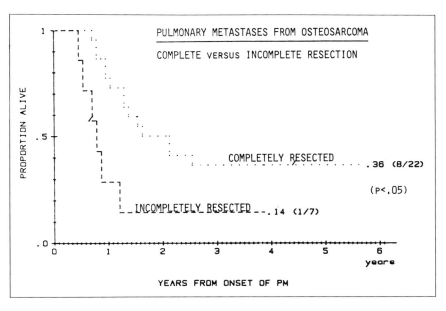

Fig. 1. Life table analysis of the overall survival of patients undergoing complete versus incomplete resection of pulmonary metastases during their first surgical exploration (see text).

Seven patients had pulmonary lesions incompletely resected during their first surgical exploration (i.e., gross residual disease or microscopic evidence of tumor at resection margins). Six of these have died with disease (fig. 1, lower curve). The only survivor had an initial median sternotomy with removal of 17 nodules from his right lung and 13 nodules from his left lung; he was rendered disease-free by a subsequent thoracotomy with resection of 3 additional nodules.

In contrast, 8 of 22 patients survived after complete resection of pulmonary lesions during their first surgical exploration, for an actuarial 5-year survival rate of 36% (fig. 1, upper curve). The difference between these groups is significant ($p < 0.05$, log rank test).

There was no significant difference in the actuarial 5-year postmetastatic survival rates according to the number of pulmonary lesions resected during the initial exploration in patients with complete resection: 33% (3 of 9 patients) after removal of solitary lesions versus 50% (2 of 4 patients) after removal of 2–5 nodules versus 33% (3 of 9 patients) after removal of 6 nodules or more.

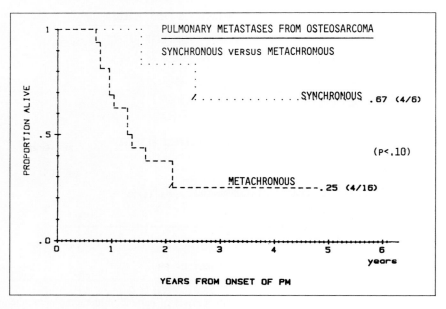

Fig. 2. Overall survival of patients with synchronous versus metachronous metastases after complete resection of metastases during their first surgical exploration (see text).

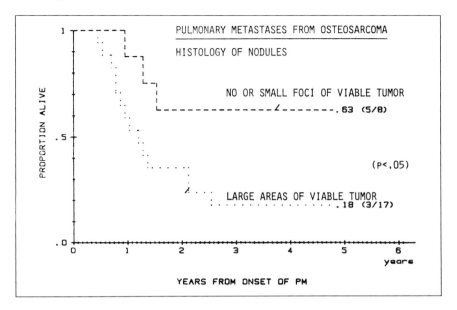

Fig. 3. Overall survival of patients whose metastases contained no or only small foci versus large areas of viable tumor (see text). Four patients undergoing thoracotomy were not evaluable in this regard.

Of the patients with complete metastasectomy at initial exploration, those with synchronous primary tumor and pulmonary metastases had a remarkably high actuarial survival rate of 67% (fig. 2, upper curve) compared with 25% in those with metachronous metastases (fig. 2, lower curve). This trend, however, is not statistically significant.

Postmetastatic chemotherapy of variable duration was performed with a variety of agents in 25 of the 29 patients undergoing thoracotomy(-ies). An attempt to classify the extent of tumor cell destruction described in the histopathological reports of resected nodules revealed virtually no or only small foci of viable tumor in 8 cases. Five of these survived with no evidence of disease (fig. 3, upper curve), in contrast to only 3 out of 17 patients with larger areas of viable tumor (fig. 3, lower curve). The corresponding survival rates are 63% and 18% respectively, and the difference is statistically significant ($p < 0.05$).

Discussion

Despite the disadvantages of a retrospective analysis, we were able to demonstrate that a long-term survival rate similar to those reported from single-institution series can be reproduced in a multicenter setting. The patients who underwent thoracotomy were treated at 14 different institutions, and there was considerable variation in surgical management as well as in the duration and regimens of postmetastatic chemotherapy.

The relatively high rate of unilateral thoracotomies indicates that there is still a potential for improvement of the results: Median sternotomy with exploration of both lungs should be the preferred initial procedure, especially in patients with more than solitary lesions on preoperative tomograms [10], since it has been repeatedly demonstrated that experienced surgeons often find more lesions during thoracotomy than previously suspected [10, 11]. It seems, therefore, that the surgical management of the (relatively rare) patients with pulmonary metastases from osteosarcoma should become more centralized at relatively few institutions in order to improve the rate of complete resections and, possibly, the long-term survival rate by a consequential and aggressive approach performed by surgeons highly specialized in pulmonary metastasectomy.

Our finding that the number of pulmonary nodules resected does not influence postmetastatic survival provided the resection was complete supports the early statement of Martini et al. [1] that pulmonary metastases of osteosarcoma should be resected whenever feasible, regardless of 'whether solitary or multiple, whether unilateral or bilateral'. Our limited experience with synchronous metastases indicates that these patients must not be excluded from metastasectomy, since their prognosis is not a priori worse than that of patients with metachronous lesions.

We have discussed the role of chemotherapy in metastatic osteosarcoma in our previous report [9]. Now that the difference in long-term survival rates between patients with large areas of viable tumor and those with no or only small foci has reached statistical significance with longer observation, we can more safely conclude that effective chemotherapy is in fact capable of improving the results. In view of the many different regimens applied in all recently published series (including this report), a prospectively controlled study of a precisely defined regimen appears highly desirable in order to refine and thereby improve the chemotherapeutic treatment of osteosarcoma metastatic to the lung.

Acknowledgement

This work was supported in part by Grant No. PTB 8350 IBCT 334 from the 'Bundesministerium für Forschung und Technologie'.

References

1   Martini, N.; Huvos, A. G.; Mike, V. et al.: Multiple pulmonary resections in the treatment of osteogenic sarcoma. Ann. thor. Surg. *12:* 271–280 (1971).

2   Goorin, A. M.; Delorey, M.; Lack, E. E. et al.: Prognostic significance of complete surgical resection of pulmonary metastases in patients with osteogenic sarcoma: analysis of 32 cases. J. clin. Oncol. *2:* 425–431 (1984).

3   Beattie, E. J.; Martini, N.; Rosen, G.: The management of pulmonary metastases in children with osteogenic sarcoma with surgical resection combined with chemotherapy. Cancer *35:* 618–621 (1975).

4   Putnam, J. B.; Roth, J. A.; Wesley, M. N. et al.: Survival following aggressive resection of pulmonary metastases from osteogenic sarcoma: analysis of prognostic factors. Ann. thorac. Surg. *36:* 516–523 (1983).

5   Rosen, G.; Huvos, A. G.; Mosende, C. et al.: Chemotherapy and thoracotomy for metastatic osteosarcoma. A model for adjuvant chemotherapy and the rationale for the timing of thoracic surgery. Cancer *41:* 841–849 (1978).

6   Rosenberg, S. A.; Flye, M. W.; Conkle, D. et al.: Treatment of osteogenic sarcoma. II. Aggressive resection of pulmonary metastases. Cancer Treat. Rep. *63:* 753–756 (1979).

7   Winkler, K.; Beron, G.; Schellong, G. et al.: Kooperative Osteosarkomstudie COSS-77: Ergebnisse nach über 4 Jahren. Klin. Pädiat. *194:* 251–256 (1982).

8   Winkler, K.; Beron, G.; Salzer-Kuntschik, M. et al.: Neoadjuvant chemotherapy for osteogenic sarcoma: results of a cooperative German/Austrian study. J. clin. Oncol. *2:* 617–624 (1984).

9   Beron, G.; Euler, A.; Winkler, K.: Pulmonary metastases from osteogenic sarcoma: complete resection and effective chemotherapy contributing to improved prognosis. Eur. Paediat. Haematol. Oncol. *2:* 77–85 (1985).

10   Johnston, M. R.: Median sternotomy for resection of pulmonary metastases. J. thorac. cardiovasc. Surg. *85:* 516–522 (1983).

11   Gürtler, K. F.; Riebel, T.; Beron, G. et al.: Vergleich von Röntgenübersichtsaufnahmen, Röntgenschichtaufnahmen und Computertomogrammen bei pulmonalen Rundherden im Kindes- und Jugendalter. Fortschr. Röntgenstr. *140:* 416–420 (1984).

Dr. med. Gerhard Beron, Abteilung für pädiatrische Hämatologie und Onkologie, Universitäts-Kinderklinik, Martinistr. 52, D-2000 Hamburg (FRG)

Contr. Oncol., vol. 30, pp. 150–159 (Karger, Basel 1988)

Treatment Results in Pulmonary Metastasized Germ Cell Tumors of the Testis

N. Niederle[a], J. Lüder[a], M. Walz[b]

[a] Innere Klinik und Poliklinik (Tumorforschung), Universitätsklinikum Essen, FRG
[b] Abteilung für Thoraxchirurgie, Universitätsklinikum Essen, FRG

Histological Classification

More than 90% of all testicular tumors are derived from immature germ cells, according to Dixon and Moore [6]. All histological classifications currently in use distinguish between seminomas and a variety of more or less immature non-seminomatous tumors, the so-called teratomas [4, 16]. Each of these histological entities can secrete specific tumor markers reflecting the course of the disease ([11, 13, 26, 37]; see table I). The most important are the glycoproteins alpha-fetoprotein

Table I. Histological classification of malignant germ cell tumors of the testis (from [4])

	β-HCG	AFP
Seminoma (S)		
Typical	(+)	−
Spermatocytic		
Teratoma		
Differentiated (TD) (mature and immature)	−	−
Malignant teratoma intermediate (MTI)	+	+
Malignant teratoma anaplastic (MTA)	+	+
Malignant teratoma trophoblastic (MTT)	+ + +	+
Combined tumors		
Seminoma and teratomas		
coexisting in the same testis	+	+
Yolk sac tumors	−	+ +

(AFP) and/or the beta unit of human chorionic gonadotropin (beta-HCG). In addition, the non-specific lactate dehydrogenase (LDH) has proven to be a useful parameter of tumor mass.

Pure seminomas constitute nearly 40% of all germ cell tumors and predominantly manifest in the 4th to 5th decade of life. The diagnosis, as a rule, is made during the early stages of the disease. For this reason, the vast majority of patients with this radiosensitive malignancy receive radiation therapy. It is rare that a cytostatic chemotherapy is indicated; therefore, the overall very good results of systemic treatment are not dealt with here [9, 22, 32].

This is not the case for non-seminomatous testicular cancer which is only slightly sensitive to radiation therapy. The social significance of this rare type of cancer, which has an incidence of 1−3 per 100,000 male residents per year, lies in the fact that it is the most common cause of death among cancer patients in the 25−34-year-old age group. The median age of our patients was 27, which agrees with data published in the literature [19, 20]. In addition, long-term investigations give evidence of an increase in the incidence of this disease.

Determination of the Stage of Disease

Suspicion of testicular cancer is usually followed by an orchidectomy. Further decisions regarding therapy depend on the results of clinical, radiologic, sonographic, serologic and operative examinations to determine the stage of disease. A variety of subdivisions has proven necessary in order to classify the stage of disease accurately and to initiate optimal therapy − that is, to insure that the patient is certainly not under- but also not overtreated [1, 20, 38]. Moreover, an accurate determination of the stage of the disease makes it easier to compare the various types of therapy studies and reach conclusions about the efficiency of individual treatment protocols.

Disseminated non-seminomatous testicular cancer, which usually means pulmonary metastases, is classified as stage III or IV according to the Essen classification [19, 34]. Since the extent of generalized metastasis formation can vary considerably, we have subdivided stage IV into A−D. In stage IV-A only minimal pulmonary metastases (< 5, diameter < 2 cm) are present. In stage IV-B patients show advanced pulmonary involvement, in stage IV-C there is additional retroperitoneal tumor invasion. In stage IV-D, besides the pulmonary metastases, extensive retroperitoneal and/or organ metastases are found.

Chemotherapy

In the last 10–15 years, enormous advances have been made in the treatment of disseminated non-seminomatous testicular cancer. They must be viewed as being largely the success of intensive cytostatic combination therapies. Among the various cytostatic drugs, vinblastine, bleomycin, cis-platinum, etoposide, ifosfamide, and, to a lesser degree, actinomycin-D, adriamycin, vincristine, and methotrexate have proven to be particularly effective individual substances.

In contrast to other centers which, following the most commonly used PVB protocol [7], recommend fixed combinations of 3 or 4 cytostatic agents given at regular intervals [21, 23, 29, 35], we prefer a sequentially alternating administration of at least 2 non-cross-resistant cytostatic combinations. A similar approach is used by the group of Newlands and Bagshawe in London [17]. This type of cytostatic administration was developed in our department in the mid-seventies in response to the pronounced heterogeneity of testicular tumor tissue. Later, it found theoretical support from Goldin et al. [10]. In any case, the current treatment of non-seminomatous testicular cancer should always be begun with expectations of a cure, even though the different stages of disease do give rise to differing prognoses (the extent of tumor is the most important prognostic factor).

Between 1978 and 1982, 115 patients were treated at the West German Tumor Center in Essen for stage IV non-seminomatous testicular cancer. Complete remissions (CR) were achieved in a total of 62% of patients, showing a direct relationship to the tumor stage and, therefore, tumor burden. The CR rate for stage IV-A was 91%, for stage IV-B and IV-C 50–70%, respectively. In the far advanced stage IV-D, the CR rate was just below 30%.

Accordingly, the median and long-term survival rates in the individual stages show statistically significant differences (fig. 1). The best results were achieved in stage IV-A with more than 90% of patients still surviving relapse-free after 4–5 years and who therefore can be considered cured. The results in stages IV-B and IV-C were decidedly worse, with survival rates of 50–60%. In stage IV-D, only about 20% of pa-

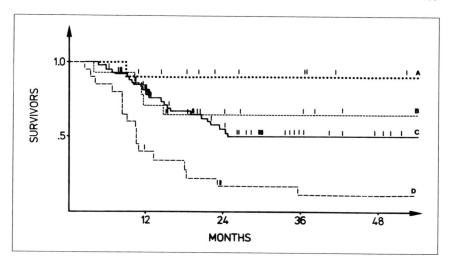

Fig. 1. Actuarial survival in stages IV A–D.

Table II. Cytostatic combinations for the treatment of non-seminomatous testicular cancer [18, 34]

Drug	Dosage	Method	Schedule
Vinblastine	0.2 mg/kg	i.v.	days 1 + 2
Bleomycin	30 E	24-h infusion	days 1 – 5
Adriamycin	60 mg/m²	i.v.	day 1
Cis-platinum	20 mg/m²	infusion	days 1 – 5
Ifosfamide	40 mg/kg	infusion	days 1 – 5
Etoposide	100 mg/m²	1-h infusion	days 1, 3, 5

tients had a chance of long-term survival. The type of combination chemotherapy, whether adriamycin/cis-platinum, vinblastine/bleomycin or etoposide/ifosfamide given as first course of therapy, has not yet been shown to influence meaningfully the median or long-term survival rates (table II, fig. 2).

Besides the stage of disease, the locations of metastases and particularly the pre-therapeutic LDH serum titers have been shown to be

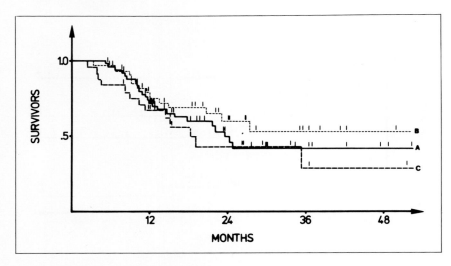

Fig. 2. Length of survival as a function of the type of first cytostatic combination.
A = vinblastine/bleomycin; B = adriamycin/cis-platinum; C = etoposide/ifosfamide or
PVB.

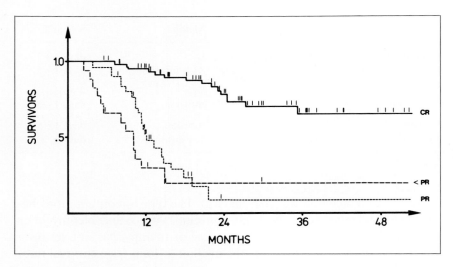

Fig. 3. Long-term survival rates as a function of the effectiveness of combination
chemotherapy. CR = complete remission; PR = partial remission; < PR = stable or
progressive disease.

significant prognostic factors in our own as well as in comprehensive investigations by others [2, 14, 27, 36]. It is, however, true for all stages of disease that the induction of complete remission significantly improves long-term survival (fig. 3). This is in contrast to partial remission (PR) induced by combination chemotherapy, which is of little benefit for the outcome of the disease: in this group of patients the median survival time was about 12 months. The few long-lasting survivals might be related to effective second- or third-line therapy or to residual mature teratomas.

Operation

Because of this poor outcome in chemotherapeutically induced PR, it has proven especially important to surgically remove residual tumor tissue, which mainly can be found in large pulmonary and, even more common, bulky retroperitoneal metastases and which generally gives rise to recurrence of disease [3, 8, 12, 15, 23].

Between 1977 and 1984, 33 patients with radiologically confirmed residual disease after chemotherapy were operated on in the Essen University Clinic for Thoracic Surgery. All patients had negative serum titer

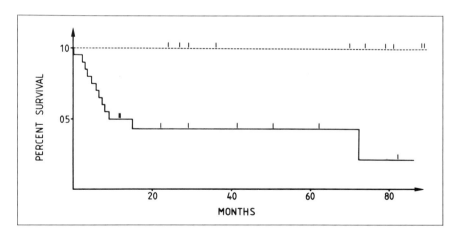

Fig. 4. Survival after surgical removal of radiologically confirmed residual tumor tissue following cytostatic chemotherapy. – – – – non vital tumor tissue found; ———— histologically confirmed vital tumor tissue.

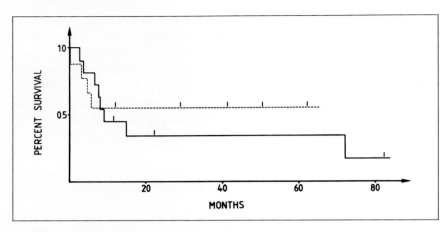

Fig. 5. Length of survival as a function of the number of surgically removed lung tumors. ——— one; — — — two or more.

values for tumor markers AFP, beta-HCG and LDH. Both single and double thoracotomies were performed. The histological examination in 10 patients showed no vital tumor tissue, and these patients have been relapse-free for an average of 4.6 years (fig. 4). Even patients with vital tumor tissue, however, benefitted from the operation. With this group of patients, the actuarial 5-year survival rate was just below 40%. For the prognosis, it proved to be of little significance whether residual tissue had to be removed from one or more sites (fig. 5) or whether this tissue was removed from one or both lungs. Whether all tumor tissue could be removed, however, proved to have a significant impact on the survival rate — as was demonstrated by the short survival of 5 patients, in whom tumor tissue could not be completely removed.

Future Directions

Between 50 and 70% of patients with disseminated non-seminomatous testicular cancer currently can be cured with the standard cytostatic chemotherapy combinations — however, only when the tumor invasion is not too extensive. In cases of extensive tumor burden (bulky disease or stage IV-D) residual tumor tissue often remains even after long-lasting chemotherapy, and here the chances of long-term survival are very definitely reduced.

In these cases it is permissible to intensify the chemotherapy and thus increase the chances of achieving complete remission and a long-term relapse-free survival rate, both of which are most important for cure [5, 25, 30]. In principle, there are two possible courses. The first is an additional increase in the dose of the most effective cytostatic agents such as cis-platinum, etoposide or ifosfamide as part of a fixed maximum combination therapy, administered at regular and short intervals [33]. And the second is the sequential or sequentially alternating administration of a variety of intensive combinations, even in the form of hybrid combinations. Many such attempts are under current investigation all over the world. With these procedures, even in advanced disease, a complete remission rate of 50−80% appears to be possible. Moreover, preliminary results indicate a relatively low relapse rate which supports hopes for a high long-term survival rate. These results might be improved by post-chemotherapy surgical removal of residual pulmonary or retroperitoneal tumor tissue.

References

1   Birch, R.; Williams, S.; Cone, A.; Einhorn, L.; Roark, P.; Turner, S.; Greco, F. A., for the Southeastern Cancer Study Group: Prognostic factors for favorable outcome in disseminated germ cell tumors. J. clin. Oncol. 4: 400−407 (1986).

2   Bosl, G. J.; Geller, N. L.; Cirrincione, C. et al.: Multivariant analysis of prognostic variables in patients with metastatic testicular cancer. Cancer Res. 43: 3403−3407 (1983).

3   Callery, C. D.; Holmes, E. C.; Vernon, S. et al.: Resection of pulmonary metastases from nonseminomatous testicular tumors. Correlation of clinical and histological features with treatment outcome. Cancer 51: 1152−1158 (1983).

4   Collins, D. H.; Pugh, R. C. B.: Classification and frequency of testicular tumours. Br. J. Urol. 36: suppl, pp. 1−12 (1964).

5   Daugaard, G.; Rørth, M.: High-dose cisplatin and VP-16 with bleomycin, in the management of advanced metastatic germ cell tumors. Eur. J. Cancer clin. Oncol. 22: 477−485 (1986).

6   Dixon, F. J.; Moore, R. A.: Tumors of the male sex organs. Atlas of tumor pathology; Sect. 8, Fasc. 31 b/32 (Armed Forces Institute of Pathology, Washington 1952).

7   Einhorn, L. H.; Donohue, J.: cis-Diamminedichloroplatinum, vinblastine and bleomycin combination chemotherapy in disseminated testicular cancer. Ann. intern. Med. 87: 293−298 (1977).

8   Einhorn, L. H.; Williams, S. D.; Mandelbaum, I.; Donohue, J. P.: Surgical resection
     in disseminated testicular cancer following chemotherapeutic cytoreduction.
     Cancer 48: 904–908 (1981).

9   Friedman, L.; Garnick, M. B.; Stomper, P. C. et al.: Therapeutic guidelines and
     results in advanced seminoma. J. clin. Oncol. 3: 1325–1332 (1985).

10   Goldie, J. H.; Coldman, A. J.; Gudauskas, G. A.: Rationale for the use of alternat-
     ing non-cross-resistant chemotherapy. Cancer Treat. Rep. 66: 439–449 (1982).

11   Heyderman, E.: Advances in pathology and immunocytochemistry. J. R. Soc. Med.
     78: suppl. 6, pp. 9–18 (1985).

12   Javadpour, N.; Ozols, R. F.; Anderson, T. et al.: A randomized trial of cytoreductive
     surgery followed by chemotherapy versus chemotherapy alone in bulky stage III
     testicular cancer with poor prognostic features. Cancer 50: 2004–2010 (1982).

13   Light, P. A.: Tumour markers in testicular cancer. J. R. Soc. Med. 78: suppl. 6,
     pp. 19–24 (1985).

14   Lippert, M. C.; Javadpour, N.: Lactic dehydrogenase in the monitoring and progno-
     sis of testicular cancer. Cancer 48: 2274–2278 (1981).

15   Logothetis, C. J.; Samuels, M. L.: Surgery in the management of stage III germinal
     cell tumors. Observations on the M. D. Anderson Hospital experience, 1971–1979.
     Cancer Treat. Rev. 11: 27–37 (1984).

16   Mostofi, F. K.; Sobin, L. H.: Histological typing of testis tumours (WHO, Genf
     1977).

17   Newlands, E. S.; Begent, R. H. J.; Rustin, G. J. S. et al.: Further advances in the
     management of malignant teratomas of the testis and other sites. Lancet i: 948–951
     (1983).

18   Niederle, N.; Scheulen, M. E.; Cremer, M. et al.: Ifosfamide in combination chemo-
     therapy for sarcomas and testicular carcinomas. Cancer Treat. Rev. 10: suppl. A,
     pp. 129–135 (1983).

19   Niederle, N.; Schütte, J.; Krischke, W. et al.: Nichtseminomatöse Hodenkarzinome
     – Behandlungsergebnisse bei hämatogener Disseminierung (Stadium IV). Verh. dt.
     Ges. inn. Med. 90: 1021–1023 (1984).

20   Niederle, N.; Seeber, S.: Nicht-seminomatöse Hodentumoren. Therapiemöglich-
     keiten und Behandlungsergebnisse bei lokoregionaler Metastasierung (Stadium II).
     Therapiewoche 34: 3311–3321 (1984).

21   Peckham, M. J.; Barrett, A.; Liew, K. et al.: The treatment of metastatic germ-cell
     testicular tumours with bleomycin, etoposide and cis-platin (BEP). Br. J. Cancer
     47: 613–619 (1983).

22   Peckham, M. J.; Horwich, A.; Hendry, W. F.: Advanced seminoma: Treatment with
     cis-platinum-based combination chemotherapy or carboplatin (JM 8). Br. J. Cancer
     52: 7–13 (1985).

23   Pizzocaro, G.; Piva, L.; Salvioni, R. et al.: Cisplatin, etoposide, bleomycin first-line
     therapy and early resection of residual tumor in far-advanced germinal testis
     cancer. Cancer 56: 2411–2415 (1985).

24   Pizzocaro, G.; Salvioni, R.; Zanoni, F. et al.: Successful treatment of good-risk dis-
     seminated testicular cancer with cisplatin, bleomycin, and reduced-dose vinblastine.
     Cancer 57: 2114–2118 (1986).

25   Samson, M. K.; Rivkin, S. E.; Jones, S. E. et al.: Dose-response and dose-survival
     advantage for high versus low-dose cisplatin combined with vinblastine and bleo-

mycin in disseminated testicular cancer. A Southwest Oncology Group study. Cancer *53:* 1029–1035 (1984).

26 Scheulen, M. E.; Niederle, N.; Bierbaum, W. et al.: Bedeutung der Tumormarker α_1-Fetoprotein und β-HCG bei der Stadieneinteilung maligner Hodentumoren. Beitr. Onkol., vol. 8, pp. 30–37 (1982).

27 Scheulen, M. E.; Pfeiffer, R.; Höffken, K. et al.: Long-term survival and prognostic factors in patients with disseminated nonseminomatous testicular cancer. Proc. Am. Soc. clin. Oncol. *3:* 163 (1984).

28 Schmidt, C. G.; Seeber, S.: Chemotherapie testikulärer Tumoren. Dt. med. Wschr. *104:* 1488–1493 (1979).

29 Schmoll, H.-J.; Diehl, V.; Hartlapp, J. et al.: PVB ± Ifosfamid bei disseminierten Hodentumoren: Ergebnisse einer prospektiv randomisierten Studie. Verh. dt. KrebsGes. *4:* 703–711 (1983).

30 Schmoll, H.-J.; Arnold, H.; Mayr, T. et al.: Platinum-ultra high dose/etoposide/ bleomycin: An effective regimen for testicular cancer with poor prognosis. Proc. Am. Soc. clin. Oncol. *3:* 163 (1984).

31 Schütte, J.; Bremer, K.; Niederle, N. et al.: Sequentiell-alternierende Chemotherapie nicht-seminomatöser Hodentumoren mit Adriamycin/Cisplatin und Bleomycin/ Vinblastin. Therapieansprechen und -versagen in Abhängigkeit von Histologie und Tumorstadium. Onkologie *6:* 16–20 (1983).

32 Schütte, J.; Niederle, N.; Scheulen, M. E. et al.: Chemotherapy of metastatic semi- noma. Br. J. Cancer *51:* 467–472 (1985).

33 Seeber, S.; Higi, M.; Niederle, N.; Schmidt, C. G.: Individualisierte Intervallverkür- zung zur Verbesserung der Induktionsbehandlung bei der Chemotherapie solider Tumoren. Dt. med. Wschr. *106:* 1741–1744 (1981).

34 Seeber, S.; Schütte, J.; Niederle, N.; Schmidt, C. G.: Neue Ergebnisse der Behand- lung metastasierter Hodentumoren im Früh- und Spätstadium. TumorDiagn. Ther. *4:* 45–54 (1983).

35 Stoter, G.; Vendrik, C. P. J.; Struyvenberg, A. et al.: Five-year survival of patients with disseminated non-seminomatous testicular cancer treated with cisplatin, vin- blastine, and bleomycin. Cancer *54:* 1521–1524 (1984).

36 Taylor, R. E.; Duncan, W.; Horn, D. B.: Lactate dehydrogenase as a marker for tes- ticular germ-cell tumours. Eur. J. Cancer clin. Oncol. *22:* 647–653 (1986).

37 Vogelzang, N. J.; Lange, P. H.; Goldman, A. et al.: Acute changes of α-fetoprotein and human chorionic gonadotropin during induction chemotherapy of germ cell tumors. Cancer Res. *42:* 4855–4861 (1982).

38 Vugrin, D.; Whitmore, W. F., Jr.; Golbey, R. B.: VAB-6 combination chemotherapy without maintenance in treatment of disseminated cancer of the testis. Cancer *51:* 211–215 (1983).

Prof. Dr. N. Niederle, Innere Universitätsklinik und Poliklinik (Tumorforschung), Hufelandstr. 55, D-4300 Essen (FRG)

Contr. Oncol., vol. 30, pp. 160–171 (Karger, Basel 1988)

Clinical Significance of Intrathoracic Manifestations of Malignant Lymphomas

M. Pfreundschuh, M. Loeffler, V. Diehl

German Hodgkin's Study Group, University Medical Clinic I, Cologne, FRG

Introduction

Whereas intrathoracic manifestations of solid tumors usually represent clinical situations which necessitate a specific therapeutic approach, intrathoracic manifestations of malignant lymphomas are generally considered part of a systemic disease that does not merit special considerations. While this might be true for the majority of cases, we would like to concentrate in this study on special situations where the localization or the extent of the disease in the thorax often requires a modification of the usual stage-adapted therapeutic approach.

Incidence and Localization of Intrathoracic Manifestations of Malignant Lymphomas

Intrathoracic Lymphadenopathy

In a prospective study Filly et al. [14] analyzed the findings in 165 untreated newly diagnosed patients with Hodgkin's disease and 136 patients with non-Hodgkin's lymphomas. The incidence and localization of the intrathoracic manifestations are shown in table I. Sixty-seven percent of the patients with Hodgkin's disease had radiographic evidence of intrathoracic disease and almost 99% of this subgroup had evidence of intrathoracic lymphadenopathy. Of 500 untreated patients with Hodgkin's disease reported to the German Hodgkin's Study Group between 1982 and 1986 (fig. 1) 50% had mediastinal lymphadenopathy and 32% had hilar involvement. The incidence of intrathoracic disease was especially high in the nodular sclerosis subgroup where 65% of the patients showed intrathoracic disease. In most cases multiple intra-thoracic lymph nodes were involved.

In patients with non-Hodgkin's lymphoma, intrathoracic disease is less common. Filly et al. [14] observed intrathoracic manifestations in

Table I. Incidence and site of intrathoracic involvement in Hodgkin's disease and non-Hodgkin's lymphomas (from [4])

	Hodgkin's disease	Non-Hodgkin's lymphomas
Intrathoracic disease	67%	44%
Anterior mediastinal	45%	14%
Tracheobronchial	44%	14%
Paratracheal	41%	14%
Bronchopulmonary	20%	10%
Subcarinal	12%	4%
Internal mammary	7%	1%
Posterior mediastinal	5%	10%
Pericardiac	2%	4%
Lung parenchyma	12%	4%
Pleura	7%	10%
Bone	3%	1%

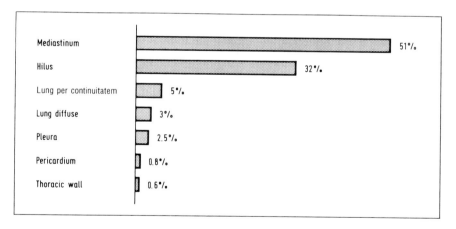

Fig. 1. Incidence of intrathoracic manifestations in 500 newly diagnosed untreated patients with Hodgkin's disease reported to the German Hodgkin's Study Group between 1982 and 1986.

40% of the cases. Involvement of a single lymph node group was observed in 30% of these cases, and 87% had radiographic evidence of intrathoracic lymphadenopathy. 'Mediastinal skipping', i.e. involvement of lymph nodes on both sides of the diaphragm without mediastinal or hilar lymphadenopathy is most often observed in the nodular lymphomas [18]. On the other hand, mediastinal involvement is rather common in 30% of cases with centrocytic lymphoma and more than half of the patients with lymphoblastic lymphoma of the T cell and unclassified type [5].

Pulmonary Parenchymal Lesions

Two cases of primary pulmonary Hodgkin's disease without lymphonodular involvement have been reported [3, 30]. However, in our experience [11] and according to others [4] this is extremely rare. Pulmonary parenchymal lesions in Hodgkin's disease were observed in our group in 40/500 newly diagnosed untreated patients (8%). This is similar to the series of Filly et al. [14] who reported an incidence of 11.6%.

Pulmonary lesions appear in two forms: 5% of the patients in our series had localized extensions of nodal disease into adjacent lung tissue (E-stage), and 3% had diffuse parenchymal infiltration representing stage IV disease according to the Ann Arbor staging classification.

In contrast to Hodgkin's disease, intraparenchymal involvement is observed in only about 4% of cases in non-Hodgkin's lymphomas [12, 14]. Up to $1/3$ of these cases are in the form of primary lymphomas of the lung, i.e. isolated lung parenchymal involvement without associated lymphonodular disease [2].

Primary Lymphoma and Pseudolymphoma of the Lung

By definition, primary lymphoma of the lung involves only lung parenchyma and (except for ipsilateral hilar lymph nodes) no other nodal or extranodal sites. Histologically, most of these cases represent lymphomas of low-grade malignancy according to the Kiel classification, and pseudolymphomas. The distinction between malignant lymphoma of the lung and pseudolymphoma may be difficult on a morphological basis [4]. Often immunohistological techniques are necessary to determine the monoclonal or polyclonal nature of the lymphoid cells. Clinically the primary lymphomas of the lung show an indolent and only slowly progressing course and may be cured by surgical removal with perhaps additional postoperative irradiation in the case of involvement of hilar nodes.

Pleural Disease

Pleural effusions are rare both in Hodgkin's and non-Hodgkin's lymphomas. Pleural disease was observed in 2.5% of the newly diagnosed patients of the German Hodgkin's Study Group. Pleural disease never appears as the only intrathoracic sign of disease in Hodgkin's disease [4], whereas isolated pleural effusions have been reported in non-Hodgkin's lymphoma [8]. The cause of the effusions may be either partial obstruction of lymphatics by hilar and/or mediastinal lymphadenopathy or direct infiltration of the pleura by the disease process. Whereas the observation that moderate uni- or bilateral effusions may resolve following radiation to the mediastinum alone [19, 39] makes obstruction a possible pathogenetic mechanism, positive cytologic findings suggest the latter. Pleural effusions, therefore, represent a diagnostic and therapeutic dilemma, as it is difficult to decide whether to manage them as E-stage or stage IV disease. If the effusions are moderate and no extension of the disease to the pleura can be detected on CT scans, patients should be treated according to the respective E-stage. Massive effusions or positive cytological findings are usually interpreted as diffuse organ involvement (stage IV) and treated as such.

Pericardiac Disease

Pericardial effusions represent diagnostic and therapeutic problems similar to those with pleural effusions. Whereas small pericardial effusions may be detected when echocardiographic examination is performed as part of the staging procedure [28], the amount of fluid rarely exceeds quantities detectable on chest roentgenograms (1%; [22]). In the series of our Hodgkin's patients pericardiac effusions were detected in only 4/500 patients (0.8%).

Endobronchial Disease

Only a few cases with endobronchial lesions as primary manifestation of the disease have been reported both for Hodgkin's disease [15] and non-Hodgkin's lymphomas [21]. A typical symptom of endobronchial disease is hemoptysis which is observed in about half the patients. In patients with Hodgkin's disease enlarged hilar lymph nodes are present radiologically in the majority of cases. Prognosis and treatment of the patients correspond to the respective clinical stage (E-stage). Endobronchial disease in non-Hodgkin's lymphomas is usually associated with widespread disease, and therefore prognosis is guarded in these patients [21].

Thoracic Wall

Involvement of the thoracic wall is rare in our series of patients with Hodgkin's disease (3/500; 0.6%). Patients are usually staged as showing extranodal manifestations of the respective stage and treated accordingly. Thoracic wall involvement often shows rapid progression and in our experience is rather resistant to chemotherapy; in most cases additional local irradiation is indicated to obtain complete remission of the thoracic wall lesion.

Mediastinal Mass of Undefined Origin

Mediastinal masses often cause diagnostic problems. Besides infectious diseases differential diagnosis includes lymphomas, thymoma and thymic carcinoma, intrathoracic germ cell tumors, carcinoids of the thymus and thymolipomas, neurogenic tumors and mesenchymal tumors. Diagnostic measures include roentgenograms, CT scans, tumor markers, bronchoscopy and mediastinoscopy. In many cases thoracotomy is necessary. Intraoperative histologic diagnosis should be pursued but is often difficult. Intraoperative immunohistological diagnosis with monoclonal antibodies might open new diagnostic possibilities. However, most of the available immunohistological techniques that are sufficiently sensitive need time-consuming amplification steps which make intraoperative diagnosis impossible. In our hands, the use of preformed complexes of biotinylated monoclonal antibodies and avidin-enzyme conjugates (e.g. avidin-alkaline phosphatase or avidin-peroxydase) results in a rapid and highly sensitive enzyme immunoassay which should be useful for intraoperative immunodiagnosis in many cases.

Treatment of Intrathoracic Manifestations of Lymphomas

Hodgkin's Lymphomas

Patients with stage I and II supradiaphragmatic disease are usually treated with extended field radiotherapy at a dose of 40 Gy. Extended field means mantle field plus paraaortic irradiation in most patients.

Some centers treat lymphocyte depleted forms with total nodal irradiation [9]. No general consensus exists as to the optimal therapy of stage IIIA. Radiotherapy is not indicated in most cases but may be justified in surgically staged patients with minimal splenic involvement or nodal involvement above the coeliac axis (III_1). In all other cases, especially in patients with massive splenic involvement or nodal involvement below the coeliac axis (III_2), combined chemo-/radiotherapy or chemotherapy alone is recommended. Patients with stage IIIB and stage IV disease are primarily treated with chemotherapy. Common chemotherapy protocols include the MOPP regimen [10], and the ABVD regimen [34]. Recent results [11, 35] suggest that a regimen of alternating cycles of MOPP/ABVD or COPP/ABVD is superior to chemotherapy with MOPP or COPP only.

Analysis of patients with stage I and II disease [13, 37, 38] revealed subgroups of patients who carry a high risk of relapse. These patients show one or more of the following risk factors: large mediastinal mass ($> 1/3$ or $1/2$ of the thoracic diameter), involvement of 3 or more lymph node regions (II_3) and high erythrocyte sedimentation rate (> 50 mm/h in stages IA and IIA; > 30 mm/h in stages IB and IIB). Whereas organ involvement per continuitatem in most cases has a negative prognostic value only if it occurs at 2 or more sites [32], there is evidence that per continuitatem involvement of the lung carries a bad prognosis even if it is unilocal [25, 33], unless the lungs are irradiated prophylactically [7]. Combined primary chemoradiotherapy is recommended in these patients.

In conclusion, as far as intrathoracic involvement is concerned, the localization and extent of intrathoracic disease has a bearing on the therapeutic approach: radiotherapy alone should not be given in stages IA–IIIA if there is a large mediastinal mass or per continuitatem involvement of the lungs, and in stages IA to IIB if intrathoracic lymphadenopathy adds to a total involvement of 3 or more lymph node areas.

In stages IIIB and IV disease the localization and extent of intrathoracic disease is of less importance for the treatment strategy, as chemotherapy is the cornerstone of therapy in these stages. If, however, bulky disease (e.g. a large mediastinal mass) is present most centers recommend additional local radiotherapy. In addition, we recommend local radiotherapy if the thoracic wall is involved, since in our experience thoracic wall involvement is relatively resistant to chemotherapy. A summary of the basic therapeutic concepts of Hodgkin's disease and recom-

Table II. Modifications of treatment strategies in Hodgkin's disease according to localization and extension of intrathoracic manifestations

Stage	Basic therapy	Recommended modification in case of		
		II$_3$	mediastinal mass	per continuitatem lung involvement
IAB	R		C + R	C + R
IIAB	R	C + R	C + R	C + R
IIIA	C or R or R + C		C + R	C + R
IIIB/IVAB	C		C + R	

C = chemotherapy
R = radiotherapy

mended modifications depending on intrathoracic findings is shown in table II.

Non-Hodgkin's Lymphomas

Treatment recommendations for non-Hodgkin's lymphomas (NHL) are shown in table III. They are based on the recommendations of the Kiel Lymphoma Group [5]. In general, localized stages of the non-Hodgkin's lymphomas of low malignancy can be cured by radiotherapy, whereas the advanced stages of most low-grade NHL do not profit from complete remissions induced by intensive polychemotherapy. These cases are usually treated with palliative chemotherapy (e.g. chlorambucil + prednisone; [24]) for the alleviation of symptoms. Some patients with advanced centroblastic-centrocytic lymphomas may profit from remission induction. The most common polychemotherapy for remission induction in low-grade NHL is the combination of cyclophosphamide, vincristine and prednisone (COP, CVP; [1]) which achieves complete remissions in more than half the patients.

In non-Hodgkin's lymphomas of high malignancy radiotherapy alone is indicated only in stage I. Stage II and advanced stages are usually treated with chemotherapy with or without additional radiotherapy. Chemotherapy protocols include combinations of cyclophosphamide, vincristine and prednisone plus doxorubicin (CHOP; [29]) or methotrexate (COMP; [40]) or bleomycin (CHOP-BLEO, [31]; BACOP,

Table III. Basic treatment recommendations for non-Hodgkin's lymphomas and possible modifications in case of intrathoracic manifestations

	I	II	III	IV
Low grade				
Lymphocytic	R*	R	C_{pal}	C_{pal}
Lymphoplasmocytic	R*	R + C_{adj}	C_{pal}	C_{pal}
Centroblastic-centrocytic	R*	R	R	$C_{rem, pal}$
Centrocytic	R*	R	C_{rem}	C_{rem}
High grade				
Centroblastic	R	C_{rem} + R	C_{rem} (+ R)	C_{rem} (+ R)
Immunoblastic	R (+ C_{rem})	C_{rem} + R**	C_{rem} (+ R)**	C_{rem} (+ R)**
Lymphoblastic	C_{rem} + R	C_{rem}**	C_{rem}**	C_{rem}**

Modifications in case of intrathoracic manifestations:
 * in case of primary lymphoma of the lung (I_E): surgery without radiotherapy possibly curative
 ** in case of mediastinal mass (T cell type): irradiation of the mediastinum recommended

C_{pal} = palliative chemotherapy
C_{rem} = intensive chemotherapy for remission induction
C_{adj} = adjuvant chemotherapy
R   = radiotherapy

[36]). Because of the different histological classification systems used, the results of the treatments can hardly be compared; complete remission rates range at about 50%. Whereas these protocols may be appropriate for centroblastic lymphomas [16], they are inadequate for the other forms of high-grade NHL. More recent protocols try to introduce as many cytotoxic drugs as possible within a short time. This can be accomplished by so-called 'hybrid' protocols or protocols using rapid alternations of two different non-cross-reacting combinations within a short time. Examples are the M-BACOD protocol [6], the ACOMLA protocol [31] and the MACOP-B protocol [23]. With these combinations the rate of complete remissions can be increased to 70–80%, but the effect on remission duration and total survival has not yet been established. Lymphoblastic lymphomas should be treated with protocols

developed for the treatment of acute lymphocytic leukemias, such as the L2 protocol [26], protocol 77-04 [27] or the BMFT protocol for the treatment of ALL [17]. Most of these protocols consist of several phases of intensive combinations of cytotoxic drugs given over several months often followed by maintenance therapy. Prophylactic treatment of the central nervous system is recommended for lymphoblastic lymphoma by most centers.

There are only a few situations with non-Hodgkin's lymphomas where localization and extent of intrathoracic involvement necessitate specific therapeutic considerations. One is in the case of primary lymphomas of the lung, the other is in the case of mediastinal mass in high-grade lymphomas (mostly T cell lymphomas).

Primary lymphomas of the lung can be cured by surgical excision alone. In the case of accompanying hilar involvement, additional radiotherapy is recommended [4]. Even though this approach seems to be straightforward it is unclear whether it represents the optimal therapy for the primary lymphomas of the lung. It should be kept in mind that most of the cases of primary lymphomas are diagnosed post festum, i.e. after definitive surgery for a putative solid tumor of the lung. There are no prospective studies comparing the surgical approach with primary irradiation. Prospective studies are needed for those cases where diagnosis can be established before thracotomy to compare the efficacy and morbidity of surgery and radiotherapy.

The second situation in NHL where intrathoracic manifestation may influence treatment strategy is the mediastinal masses in high-grade lymphomas of the T cell type. Lymphoblastic lymphomas of the T cell type are seen in 80% of children with a mediastinal mass, in adults in 55% [30]. The experience of several groups [17] shows that these patients are prone to relapse in the site of the mediastinal mass. Preliminary observations suggest that additional radiotherapy to the mediastinum after achieving complete remission with chemotherapy may prolong the remission duration. The effect of this measure on survival, however, remains to be determined.

Acknowledgement

We would like to thank Mrs. H. Nisters-Backes and Mrs. K. Smith for the statistical analysis.

References

1 Bagley, C. M.; De Vita, V. T.; Berard, C. W.; Canellos, G. P.: Advanced lymphosarcoma. Intensive cyclical combination of advanced diffuse histiocytic lymphoma. Am. J. Med. *76:* 227–234 (1972).

2 Balikian, J. P.; Hermann, P. G.: Non-Hodgkin lymphoma of the lungs. Radiology *132:* 569–576 (1979).

3 Ball, D. G.; Herman, T. E.; Variakojis, D.; Nachman, J.: Primary pulmonary Hodgkin's disease. Arch. intern. Med. *142:* 1941–1943 (1982).

4 Blank, N.; Castellino, R. A.: The intrathoracic manifestations of the malignant lymphomas and the leukemias. Semin. Roentgenol. *15:* 227–245 (1980).

5 Brittinger, G.; Meusers, P.; Musshoff, K.; Gyenes, T.: Non-Hodgkin-Lymphome und Plasmozytom, in: Schmidt, Gross, Klinische Onkologie, pp. 41.1–41.71 (Thieme, Stuttgart 1985).

6 Canellos, G. P.; Skarin, A. T.; Rosenthal, D. S. et al.: Methotrexate as a single agent and in combination chemotherapy for the treatment of non-Hodgkin's lymphoma of unfavourable histology. Cancer Treat, Rep. *65:* suppl. 1, pp. 125–129 (1981).

7 Carmel, R. J.; Kaplan, H. S.: Mantle irradiation in Hodgkin's disease. Cancer *37:* 2813–2821 (1976).

8 Castellino, R. A.; Bellani, F. F.; Gasparini, M. et al.: Radiographic findings in previously untreated children with non-Hodgkin's lymphoma. Radiology *117:* 657–663 (1975).

9 De Vita, V. T.; Jaffe, E. S.; Hellman, S.: Hodgkin's disease and the non-Hodgkin's lymphomas; in: De Vita, Hellman, Rosenberg, Cancer: Principles and practice of oncology, pp. 1623–1709 (Lippincott, Philadelphia 1985).

10 De Vita, V. T.; Serpick, A.: Combination chemotherapy in the treatment of advanced Hodgkin's disease. Proc. Am. Ass. Cancer Res. *8:* 13 (1967).

11 Diehl, V.; Pfreundschuh, M.; Hauser, F. E. et al.: Zwischenergebnisse der Therapiestudien HD 1, HD 2 und HD 3 der Deutschen Hodgkin-Studiengruppe. Med. Klinik *1:* 1–6 (1986).

12 Dunnick, N. R.; Parker, B. R.; Castellino, R. A.: Rapid onset of pulmonary infiltration due to histiocytic lymphoma. Radiology *118:* 281–285 (1976).

13 Ferrant, A.; Hamoir, V.; Binon, J. et al.: Combined modality therapy for mediastinal Hodgkin's disease. Prognostic significance of constitutional symptoms and size of disease. Cancer *55:* 317–322 (1985).

14 Filly, R.; Blank, N.; Castellino, R. A.: Radiographic distribution of intrathoracic disease in previously untreated patients with Hodgkin's disease and non-Hodgkin's lymphoma. Radiology *120:* 277–281 (1976).

15 Harper, P. G.; Fisher, C.; McLennan, K.; Souhame, R. L.: Presentation of Hodgkin's disease as an endobronchial lesion. Cancer *53:* 147–150 (1982).

16 Heinz, R.; Neumann, E.; Aiginger, P. et al.: CHOP first-line treatment in NHL with unfavourable prognosis — evaluation of therapeutic response and factors influencing prognosis. Blut *50:* 267–276 (1985).

17 Hoelzer, D.; Thiel, E.; Löffler, H. et al.: Intensified therapy in acute leukemia in adults. Blood *64:* 38–47 (1984).

18 Jones, S. E.: Clinical features and course of the non-Hodgkin's lymphomas. Clin. Haematol. *3:* 131–160 (1974).

19 Kaplan, H. S.: Hodgkin's Disease. (Harvard University Press, Cambridge, Mass. 1972).

20 Kern, W. H.; Crepean, A. G.; Jones, J. C.: Primary Hodgkin's disease of the lung. Cancer *14:* 1151–1165 (1961).

21 Kilgore, T. L.; Chasen, M. H.: Endobronchial non-Hodgkin's lymphoma. Chest *84:* 58–61 (1983).

22 Klatte, E. C.; Yardley, J.; Smith, E. B. et al.: The pulmonary manifestations and complications of leukemia. Am. J. Roentg. *89:* 598–605 (1963).

23 Klimo, P.; Connors, J. M.: MACOP-B chemotherapy for the treatment of diffuse large-cell lymphoma. Ann. Intern. Med. *102:* 596–602 (1985).

24 Knospe, W. H.; Loeb, V.; Huguley, C. M.: Biweekly chlorambucil treatment of chronic lymphocytic leukemia. Cancer *33:* 555–562 (1974).

25 Levi, J. A.; Wiernik, P. H.: Limited extranodal Hodgkin's disease. Cancer *39:* 2158–2163 (1977).

26 Levine, A. M.; Forman, P. R.; Meyer, S. C. et al.: Successful therapy of convoluted T-lymphoblastic lymphoma in the adult. Blood *61:* 92–98 (1983).

27 Magrath, I. T.; Janus, C.; Edwards, B. K. et al.: An effective treatment for both un-differentiated (including Burkitt's) lymphomas and lymphoblastic lymphomas in children and young adults. Blood *63:* 1102–1111 (1984).

28 Markiewicz, W.; Glatstein, E.; London, E. J. et al.: Echocardiographic detection of pericardial effusion and pericardial thickening in malignant lymphoma. Radiology *123:* 161–164 (1977).

29 McKelvey, E. M.; Gottlieb, J. A.; Wilson, H. E. et al.: Hydroxyldaunomycin (adria-mycin) combination chemotherapy in malignant lymphoma. Cancer *38:* 1484–1493 (1976).

30 Müller-Weihrich, S.; Henze, G.; Jobke, A. et al.: BFM-Studie 1975–1981 zur Be-handlung der Non-Hodgkin-Lymphome hoher Malignität bei Kindern und Jugend-lichen. Klin. Pädiat. *194:* 219–225 (1982).

31 Newcomer, L. N.; Cadman, E. C.; Nerenberg, M. L. et al.: Randomized study com-paring doxorubicin, cyclophosphamide, vincristine, methotrexate with leucovorin rescue, and cytarabine (ACOMLA) with cyclophosphamide, doxorubicin, vincris-tine, prednisone and bleomycin (CHOP-B) in the treatment of diffuse histiocytic lymphoma. Cancer Treat. Rep. *66:* 1279–1284 (1982).

32 Pillai, G. N.; Hagemeister, F. B.; Velasquez, W. S. et al.: Prognostic factors for stage IV Hodgkin's disease treated with MOPP, with or without bleomycin. Cancer *55:* 691–697 (1985).

33 Rosenberg, S. A.; Kaplan, H. S.; Glatstein, E. J.; Portlock, C. S.: Combined modal-ity therapy for Hodgkin's disease. Cancer *42:* 991–999 (1978).

34 Santoro, A.; Bonfante, V.; Bonnadonna, G.: Salvage chemotherapy with ABVD in MOPP-resistant Hodgkin's disease. Ann. intern. Med. *96:* 139–143 (1982).

35 Santoro, A.; Bonnadonna, G.; Bonfante, V.; Valaguss, P.: Alternating drug combi-nations in the treatment of advanced Hodgkin's disease. New Engl. J. Med. *306:* 770–774 (1982).

36 Schein, P. S.; De Vita, V. T.; Hubbard, B. A. et al.: Bleomycin, adriamycin, cyclo-phosphamide, vincristine, and prednisone (BACOP) combination chemotherapy in the treatment of advanced diffuse histiocytic lymphoma. Ann. intern. Med. *85:* 417–422 (1976).

37   Tubiana, M.; Henry-Amar, M.; Hayat, M. et al.: Prognostic significance of the number of involved areas in the early stages of Hodgkin's disease. Cancer *54:* 885–894 (1984).
38   Tubiana, M.; Henry-Amar, M.; van der Werf-Messing, B. et al.: A multivariate analysis of prognostic factors in early stage Hodgkin's disease. Int. J. Radiat. Oncol. Biol. Phys. *11:* 23–30 (1985).
39   Weick, J. K.; Kiely, J. M.; Harrison, F. G. et al.: Pleural effusions in lymphoma. Cancer *31:* 848–853 (1973).
40   Ziegler, J. L.; Magrat, I. T.; Deisseraoth, A. B. et al.: Combined modality treatment of Burkitt's lymphoma. Cancer Treat. Rep. *62:* 2031–2034 (1978).

Dr. med. M. Pfreundschuh, German Hodgkin's Study Group, Med. Univ.-Klinik I, Josef-Stelzmann-Straße 9, D-5000 Köln 41 (FRG)

Contr. Oncol., vol. 30, pp. 172–180 (Karger, Basel 1988)

Pulmonary Metastases in Gynecological Cancer

M. Kaufmann, H. Schmid, F. Kubli

University Hospital, Department of Obstetrics and Gynecology, University of Heidelberg, FRG

Introduction

The lung and pleura together constitute the most frequent site of distant metastases in cancer patients. However, in general, in gynecological carcinomas pulmonary metastases are not often seen.

Early diagnosis of pulmonary metastases is important, because if diagnosed at an asymptomatic stage, the results are more favorable than when symptoms are evident.

Diagnosis includes conventional X-ray, tomography, computer tomography, and biopsies for cytological and histological examinations.

During the last few decades great advances in the treatment of pulmonary metastases have been made. These mainly include surgery and first and foremost chemo- or hormonotherapy. Radiation therapy seems to be of marginal benefit.

The value of adjuvant systemic treatment in gyneological cancer remains unclear to date with respect to preventing pulmonary metastases.

Frequency and Time of Occurrence

The frequency of pulmonary metastases in different gynecological malignancies is shown in table I. Pulmonary metastases are most common in choriocarcinomas with rates up to 80%, whereas lung metastases occur less frequently in ovary, endometrium, and cervical cancer. Kerr and Cadman [8], in an analysis from 1966 to 1975, reported that

Table I. Frequency of pulmonary metastases in gynecological malignancies

Primary tumor site	%	Author (reference)	
Cervix (adeno carcinoma)	20.0	Sostman and Matthey	[17]
(squamous cell carcinoma)	4.0	Sostman and Matthey	[17]
	9.0	Tellis and Beechler	[19]
Endometrium	26.0	Yoonessi et al.	[22]
	16.0	Sieber	[14]
Ovary	21.3	Smith et al.	[16]
	44.5	Kerr and Cadman	[8]
Choriocarcinoma	80.0	Elston	[4]
	67.0	Tomoda et al.	[20]

Table II. Pulmonary metastases in cervical cancer (retrospective analysis 1970–1975), Tellis and Beechler [19]; frequency: 22/243 patients (= 9%)

Stage (FIGO)	% pulmonary metastases	Mean recurrence-free interval (months)
I	4.2	39.0
II	13.0	37.3
III	7.4	18.0
IV	57.0	<1.0

pulmonary metastases were found in 15% (53 patients) in ovarian carcinomas at the time of diagnosis. In 30% lung metastases were developed later (106 patients).

In a retrospective analysis from 1970 to 1975, Tellis and Beechler [19] registered in 243 cervical carcinomas a stage-related occurrence rate of pulmonary metastases combined with different recurrence-free intervals. Advanced stages were directly correlated with increased rates of metastases and shorter latent periods (table II).

In endometrium cancer, autopsy reports (time period 1930–1971) showed pulmonary metastases in 26% out of 398 patients, liver as well as bone metastases in 8% (Yoonessi et al. [22]). A more recent retrospective analysis (time period 1930–1980) of 263 autopsies represents lung metastases in 16%, pleural metastases in 10%, liver metastases in 17%, and bone involvement in 14% [14]. Ballon et al. [2] diagnosed that 2.3%

(= 33/1434) of women with endometrial carcinoma developed pulmonary metastases.

Therapy

Surgical Treatment

Only a small fraction of gynecological cancer patients are candi-
dates for resection of pulmonary metastases. Very few series of selected
cases are reported [3, 5, 6, 12, 15, 20, 21]. Table III demonstrates as an
example latent periods of the selected patients for pulmonary resection.
Of 15 women with different primary tumor sites treated by pulmonary
surgery between 1943 and 1982, 36% had a 5-year survival and 26% a
10-year survival. Mountain et al. [11] noted a 5-year actual survival of
19% (median survival 27 months) in 20 cervical cancer patients following resection of pulmonary metastases out of 159 treated cancer patients
with various tumor histologies, whereas data from Morrow et al. [10]
could show only 8% of patients with 5-year survival (18 surgically
treated patients out of 125).

Wang et al. [21] reported promising surgical treatment results with
pulmonary metastases even in 29 chemoresistant choriocarcinomas (age
23 – 52 years) during 1976 – 1980. In total, 17 women survived (3 for 1 – 3
years, 5 for 3 – 5 years, 3 for 5 – 10 years and 6 over 10 years). Of the
12 patients who died, 8 had brain metastases, 2 had gastrointestinal
tract hemorrhage and septicemia, 1 had respiratory failure and 1 case
was unknown.

Table III. Pulmonary resection in gynecological cancer patients and latent period; time
period 1943–1982, Boston; Fuller et al. [5]

Primary tumor site	n	Latent period (months)
Cervix	6	14, 24, 28, 34, 68, 96
Endometrium	3	55, 81, 110
Ovary	2	70, 108
Gestational trophoblast tumors	2	1, 2
Sarcoma	2	32, unknown
Total	15	

There is no doubt that surgical treatment of pulmonary metastases requires certain minimal criteria before undergoing such aggressive procedures [5, 6, 18].

These include the following options:

1. Patient in ensured good physiological condition for the planned resection;

2. local control of the primary tumor or complete removal;

3. no further distant metastases;

4. all pulmonary metastases are resectable (e. g. isolated unilateral metastases);

5. in choriocarcinomas: β-HCG titer < 1,000 mlU/ml;

6. prognostic factors have to be considered (e. g. tumor type, disease-free interval, number and location of metastases, tumor doubling time);

7. consent of the patient.

Prognostic Factors

Some clinical prognostic factors are known which should be taken into account to plan individualized treatment.

Table IV demonstrates prognosis dependent on the extent of disease in choriocarcinomas. Survival is clearly combined with the number and localization of metastases. This also can be demonstrated in ovarian cancer patients (table V, VI).

In our own series, however, patients with pleural effusions showed the best survival rates compared to the data demonstrated by Kerr and Cadman [8].

Table IV. Pulmonary resection for pulmonary metastases in choriocarcinomas in relation to the extension of metastases

Author (reference)	Extension of metastases	n	Prognosis	
			survived	died
Tomoda et al. [20]	bilateral	2	0	2
	unilateral	19	15	4
Wang et al. [21]	solitary	23	17	6
	multiple	6	0	6

Table V. Metastases to the chest and survival of patients with ovarian cancer* (Kerr and Cadman [8]); n = 159

Main tumor site	n	5-year survival (%)
Pleural effusion	64	2.6
Parenchymal	44	14.8
Multiple	46	6.5

* 5 patients had other isolated lesions.

Table VI. Pulmonary metastases and survival of patients with ovarian cancer (University Hospital, Heidelberg); time period 1980–1985

Tumor site	Survived (n)	Time (years)		
		1	2	5
Pleural effusion	36	32	30	4
Parenchymal				
Isolated	9	9	3	0
Multiple	14	0	0	0
Multiple metastases plus lung	34	0	0	0
Total	93	41	33	4

Chemotherapy

Recent reports demonstrate especially in non-pretreated gynecological squamous cell carcinomas encouraging data for systemic treatment [7]. Hormone sensitivity of endometrium cancer and therefore effectiveness of endocrine therapy is well known [1, 7]. Therapy results in gynecological cancer patients with lung metastases, which were achieved at our institution with cytotoxic or endocrine drugs are demonstrated in table VII.

Cis-platinum combination schedules in squamous cell carcinomas gave the best results. Duration of remissions (CR, PR) ranged between 4 and 14 months. Hormonal treatment in endometrium cancer showed even longer lasting remissions. These data were compared with those

Table VII. Chemotherapy results in pulmonary metastases of gynecological cancer (University Hospital, Heidelberg)

Primary tumor site	n	Chemotherapy	Result	Duration (months)
Cervix	2	CIS/VDS	1 CR, 1 PR	6, 8
	1	CIS/IFO	1 PR	4
	1	CIS/BLEO	1 NC	4
	1	BCNU/5 FU	1 NC	20
Endometrium	3	FEC	2 PR, 1 P	12, 14, —
	1	NOSTE	1 NC	3 +
	6	HD-MPA	2 CR	22 +
			1 PR	16
			2 NC	8
			1 P	—
Vulva	1	CIS/VDS	1 PR	4
	1	NOSTE	1 P	—
Sarcoma	1	CIS/VDS	1 CR	14
	1	CYVADIC	1 CR	12

Abbreviations see p. 179

obtained in older series without systemic therapy, if pulmonary involvement of gynecological carcinomas was diagnosed (table VIII). For all tumor sites, systemically treated patients showed longer survival compared to untreated women.

Sessa et al. [13] reported 6 remissions (2 CR, 4 PR) in cervical cancer with lung metastases, which lasted between 5.5 and 12 months.

Chemosensitivity, which is well-known in choriocarcinomas [9] could also be demonstrated in patients treated at our institution (table IX). Mean gained survival times were 75 + months for low-risk and 66 + months for medium-risk women.

Conclusions

In gynecological cancer pulmonary metastases seldom occur, with the exception of choriocarcinomas.

Table VIII. Pulmonary metastases and survival in untreated and treated patients with gynecological cancer (University Hospital, Heidelberg)

Primary tumor site	n	Age*	Pulmonary metastases, latent period (months)*	Treatment	Survival since treatment (months)*
Cervix	11	66	12.4	—	2.7
	4	65	9.0	Bromocriptin	3.0
	5	42	17.2	CHT	13.4
Endometrium	2	69	0	—	2.0
	6	62	22.1	HD-MPA	13.7 (+)
	4	54	3.3	CHT	21.8
Ovary	2	59	18	—	4
(recurrence)	2	58	24	CHT	5
Vulva	2	62	0	—	2.5
	2	66	67.0	CHT	3.5 (+)
Sarcoma	2	46	13.0	CHT	39.0
Gestational trophoblastic tumors	6	36	6.0	CHT	71.0 (+)

* Mean
Abbrevations see p. 179

Table IX. Pulmonary metastases and survival in patients with gestational choriocarcinoma (University Hospital, Heidelberg)

Risk group*	n	Chemotherapy	Result	Mean survival (months)
Low risk	4	1 MTX 2 MTX, Act. D 1 Act. D	4 CR	75 +
Medium risk	2	1 MTX/Act. D/VP-16 1 MTX/Act. D	2 CR	66 +

* Classification criteria: β-HCG (mIU/ml) titer: low risk < 40,000; medium risk > 40,000; duration of symptoms: low risk < 4 months; medium risk > 4 months
Abbreviations see p. 179

Various criteria, including the various prognostic factors, have to be considered in selecting those patients who will benefit from surgical resection, chemotherapy or endocrine treatment alone or in combination.

A comparison of a historic control group of 17 untreated and 31 systemically treated women with pulmonary metastases showed better survival for the therapy group at our institution.

List of Abbreviations

Act. D	actinomycin D
BCNU	carmustin
BLEO	bleomycin
CHT	chemotherapy
CIS	cis-platinum
CR	complete remission
CTX	cyclophosphamide
CYVADIC	cyclophosphamide/vincristine/adriamycin/DTIC
FEC	5-fluorouracil/epirubicin/cyclophosphamide
5FU	5-fluorouracil
HD-MPA	high-dose medroxyprogesterone acetate
IFO	ifosfamide
L-PAM	L-phenylalanine-mustard
MTX	methotrexate
NC	no change
NOSTE	mitoxantrone/prednimustine
P	progression
PR	partial remission
VDS	vindesine
VP-16	etoposid

References

1 Aalders, J. G.; Abeler, V.; Kolstad, P.: Recurrent adenocarcinoma of the endometrium: A clinical and histopathological study of 379 patients. Gynecol. Oncol. *17:* 85–103 (1984).

2 Ballon, S. C.; Berman, M. L.; Donaldson, R. C. et al.: Pulmonary metastases of endometrial carcinoma. Gynecol. Oncol. *7:* 56–65 (1979).

3 Braude, S.; Thompson, P. J.: Solitary pulmonary metastases in carcinoma of the cervix. Thorax *38:* 953–954 (1983).

4 Elston, C. W.: J. clin. Path. *10:* suppl., pp. 111–113 (1977).

5 Fuller, A. F.; Scannell, J. G.; Wilkins, E. W.: Pulmonary resection for metastases from gynecologic cancers: Massachusetts General Hospital experience, 1943–1982. Gynecol. Oncol. *22:* 174–180 (1985).

6   Gallousis, S.: Isolated lung metastases from pelvic malignancies. Gynecol. Oncol. *7:* 206–214 (1979).

7   Kaufmann, M.; Schmid, H.: Cytostatika- und Hormontherapie beim Cervix- und Corpus-Carcinom. Onkol. Forum *2:* 10–15 (1985).

8   Kerr, V. E.; Cadman, E. D.: Pulmonary metastases in ovarian cancer. Cancer *56:* 1209–1213 (1985).

9   Lurain, J. R.; Brewer, J. I.: Treatment of high-risk gestational trophoblastic disease with methotrexate, actinomycin D and cyclophosphamide chemotherapy. Obstet. Gynec., N. Y. *65:* 830–836 (1985).

10 Morrow, C. E.; Vassilopoulos, P.; Grage, T. B.: Surgical resection for metastatic neoplasms of the lung. Cancer *45:* 2981–2985 (1981).

11 Mountain, C. F.; Khalil, K. G.; Hermes, K. E.; Frazier, O. H.: The contribution of surgery to the management of carcinomatous pulmonary metastases. Cancer *41:* 833–840 (1978).

12 Saitoh, K.; Harada, K.; Nakayama, H. et al.: Role of thoracotomy in pulmonary metastases from gestational choriocarcinoma. J. thorac. cardiovasc. Surg. *85:* 815–820 (1983).

13 Sessa, C.; Bolis, G.; Colombo, N. et al.: Untreated lung metastases of cervical cancer: Results of three chemotherapy regimens (Abstract). UICC Lausanne (1981).

14 Sieber, M.: Metastasierung des Endometriumcarcinoms: Analyse pathoanatomischer Befunde und klinische Daten an 263 obduzierten Patientinnen. Thesis, University of Heidelberg (1982).

15 Sink, J. D.; Hammond, C. B.; Young, W. G.: Pulmonary resection in the management of metastases from gestational choriocarcinoma. J. thorac. cardiovasc. Surg. *81:* 830–834 (1981).

16 Smith, J. P.; Day, T. G.: Review of ovarian cancer at the University of Texas Systems Cancer Center, M. D. Anderson Hospital and Tumor Institute. Am. J. Obstet. Gynec. *135:* 984–993 (1979).

17 Sostman, H. D.; Matthay, R. A.: Thoracic metastases from cervical carcinoma: Current status. Investve Radiol. *15:* 113–116 (1980).

18 Takita, H.; Edgerton, F.; Karakousis, C. et al.: Surgical management of metastases to the lung. Surgery Gynec. Obstet. *152:* 191–194 (1981).

19 Tellis, C. J.; Beechler, C. R.: Pulmonary metastasis of carcinoma of the cervix: A retrospective study. Cancer *49:* 1705–1709 (1982).

20 Tomoda, Y.; Arii, Y.; Kaseki, S. et al.: Surgical indications for resection in pulmonary metastasis of choriocarcinoma. Cancer *46:* 2723–2730 (1980).

21 Wang, Y.; Song, H.; Xia, Z.; Sun, C.: Drug resistant pulmonary choriocarcinoma metastasis treated by lobectomy: Report of 29 cases. Chin. med. J. *93:* 758–766 (1980).

22 Yoonessi, M.; Anderson, D. G.; Morley, G. W.: Endometrial carcinoma. Causes of death and sites of treatment failure. Cancer *43:* 1944–1950 (1979).

Priv.-Doz. Dr. med. Manfred Kaufmann, Universitäts-Frauenklinik, Voßstr. 9, D-6900 Heidelberg 1 (FRG)

Contr. Oncol., vol. 30, pp. 181–185 (Karger, Basel 1988)

The Treatment of Breast Cancer Lung Metastases

R. Herrmann

Medizinische Klinik und Poliklinik, Universitätsklinikum Rudolf Virchow, Standort Charlottenburg, Berlin

In end-stage breast cancer the lung is the most commonly involved metastatic site (table I). This is not the case at the time when metastases are first detected (table II). In this situation it makes no difference whether metastases are detected at the time of the original diagnosis or following a disease-free interval.

Table I. Breast cancer metastatic sites at autopsy (%) (from Lee [6])

Metastatic site	%
Lungs	71
Bones	71
Lymph nodes	67
Liver	62
Pleura	50

Table II. Breast cancer – initial metastatic sites (%) [7]

Metastatic site	%
Bone	40 – 60
Lungs	15 – 22
Pleura	10 – 14
Soft tissue	7 – 15
Liver	5 – 15

The histologic subtype is the only proven risk factor for the development of lung metastases in breast cancer [4]. The chances are significantly higher with ductal carcinoma as compared to lobular carcinoma. The time from the first diagnosis is apparently not important. Even after years or decades lung metastases may develop.

Diagnostic Approaches

In patients with a history of breast cancer a solitary lesion on a chest X-ray is a special diagnostic problem.

Cahan et al. [1] detected breast cancer metastases in only 32% of 72 patients. In 60% the cause turned out to be a primary lung cancer. This observation is consistent with a Danish study where the risk of lung cancer was significantly higher in patients with a history of breast cancer [3]. Solitary nodular metastases are found only in 11% of all patients with lung metastases (table III). Multiple nodules in both lungs are much more common. AP and lateral chest X-rays will be diagnostic in most cases. Only rarely conventional tomography or computerized

Table III. Distribution of types of pulmonary metastases (%) in breast cancer [5]

Metastasis	%
Nodular	
Solitary	11
Multiple	42
Lymphangitic	52
Endobronchial	9

Table IV. Differential diagnosis of interstitial pulmonary infiltrates in breast cancer

Lymphangitic spread
Pneumonia
Radiation sequela
Chemotherapy sequela
Fibrosis of other causes
Granulomatous diseases

tomography will be necessary. With the history of breast cancer and the typical X-ray it will not be difficult to make a diagnosis. Nevertheless, other causes that could be responsible should always be taken into consideration, i.e. multiple pulmonary infarctions.

It can be much more difficult to diagnose lymphangitic lung involvement. In this situation the acute onset — fever, leukocytosis and rapid progression — can mimic pneumonia [10]. Several other diseases should be excluded (table IV).

Treatment

For therapeutic purposes the following situations should be separately considered:
- Isolated solitary nodule without other manifestations
- multiple nodules,
- lymphangiosis.

If no other manifestations of breast cancer can be detected, an isolated pulmonary nodule should be surgically removed. If this turns out to be a metastasis of breast cancer, there may be a small chance for long-term survival (table V). Similar to the situation in colon cancer, there is a correlation between the relapse-free interval and prognosis following operation. It is not known whether or not this operation should be followed by adjuvant chemotherapy. Since surgical treatment alone may induce long-term remissions, it seems likely that adjuvant chemotherapy in premenopausal women may have a beneficial effect on the relapse-free interval in the overall group. Whether surgical treatment is superior to chemotherapy and/or hormonal therapy or no treatment at all cannot be determined. Because of uncertainties in the diagnosis a surgical approach is absolutely necessary.

Table V. Long-term results following surgical removal of a solitary lung metastasis in breast cancer

5-year disease-free survival	References
14%	[9]
15%	[8]
31% (19% no evidence of disease)	[1]

Patients with multiple nodular lung metastases will generally receive systemic treatment. There are no studies to determine whether in asymptomatic patients with a small tumor volume the treatment can be withheld for some time to be able to observe the natural course of the disease. The type of the systemic treatment to be administered depends on the hormone receptor status of the tumor. If the receptor content is high or unknown a hormonal treatment is indicated. Since breast cancer is such a heterogenous disease the results of chemotherapy of nodular lung metastases can only be reported relative to the results of other metastatic sites. According to a Southeastern Cancer Study Group study the likelihood of response is similar to the one seen with loco-regional recurrences and bone metastases [11]. Response rates with the CAF regimen (cyclophosphamide, adriamycin, 5-fluorouracil) are in the range of 60–70%. These sites are the less aggressive ones. On the other hand, liver metastases and lymphangitic lung metastases or pleural manifestations are prognostically worse. These sites also show lower response rates. In addition, the duration of remissions is shorter. It is likely that the existence of liver metastases indicates a more advanced stage of the disease, which is known to poorly respond to any treatment. Also, measurability of tumor parameters is much easier with lung metastases as compared to liver metastases.

Patients with a lymphangitic spread to the lungs should receive primary combination chemotherapy without delay. Especially if pulmonary function is impaired a regimen should be used which is likely to produce a high remission rate. If the hormone receptor status is positive, hormone treatment should be started simultaneously. The aim of the treatment must be to rapidly decrease tumor burden and improve pulmonary function. In addition, some authors recommend glucocorticoids [2]. Other supportive measures such as oxygen, diuretics and digoxin may be helpful. In these situations with respiratory insufficiency even small pleural effusions should be tapped if a chemotherapy-induced remission seems to be possible.

There is no indication for radiotherapy of lung metastases in breast cancer.

Except for a few situations that have been mentioned, lung metastases from breast cancer require no special management. In most cases they are just one of many manifestations of this disease. Prognostically nodulary lung metastases are favorable while lymphangitic spread to the lungs is rather unfavorable.

References

1   Cahan, W. G.; Castro, E. B.: Significance of a solitary lung shadow in patients with breast cancer. Ann. Surg. *181:* 137–143 (1975).

2   Coombes, R. C.: Medical complications of advanced breast cancer; in Coombes, Powles, Ford et al., Breast cancer management, pp. 205–226 (Academic Press, London 1981).

3   Ewertz, M.; Mouridsen, H. T.: Second cancer following cancer of the female breast in Denmark, 1943–1980. Natn. Cancer Inst. Monogr. *68:* 325–329 (1985).

4   Harris, M.; Howell, A.; Chrissohou, M. et al.: A comparison of the metastatic pattern of infiltrating lobular and infiltrating duct carcinoma of the breast. Br. J. Cancer *50:* 23–30 (1984).

5   Kreisman, H.; Wolkove, N.; Schwartz Finkelstein, H.; et al.: Breast cancer and thoracic metastases: review of 119 patients. Thorax *38:* 175–179 (1983).

6   Lee, Y. T.: Breast carcinoma: Pattern of metastasis at autopsy. J. surg. Oncol. *23:* 175–180 (1983).

7   Lee, Y. T.: Breast carcinoma: Pattern of recurrence and metastasis after mastectomy. Am. J. clin. Oncol. *7:* 443–449 (1984).

8   McCormack, P. M.; Bains, M. S.; Beattie, J. R. et al.: Pulmonary resection in metastatic carcinoma. Chest *73:* 163–166 (1978).

9   Mountain, C. F.; Khalil, K. G.; Hermes, K. E. et al.: The contributions of surgery to the management of carcinomatous pulmonary metastases. Cancer *41:* 833–840 (1978).

10 Nixon, D. W.; Shlaer, S. M.: Fulminant lung metastases from cancer of the breast. Med. Pediat. Oncol. *9:* 381–385 (1981).

11 Smalley, R. V.; Bartolucci, A. A.; Moore, M. et al.: Southeastern Cancer Study Group: Breast cancer studies 1972–1982. Int. J. Radiat. Oncol. Biol. Phys. *9:* 1867–1874 (1983).

Prof. Dr. R. Herrmann, Medizinische Klinik und Polikinik,
Universitätsklinikum Rudolf Virchow, Standort Charlottenburg,
Spandauer Damm 130, D-1000 Berlin 19

Contr. Oncol., vol. 30, pp. 186–194 (Karger, Basel 1988)

Lung Metastases from Gastrointestinal Tumors

H. Flechtner, W. Queißer

Onkologisches Zentrum, Klinikum Mannheim, Fakultät für klinische Medizin der Universität Heidelberg, FRG

Introduction

Today gastrointestinal malignancies cause about 40% of all cancer deaths in the population of the FRG [43]. Mainly three tumors contribute to this figure: gastric cancer, cancer of the colon and cancer of the rectum [19]. Next in importance are pancreatic and esophageal cancer. If not surgically cured, the course of the disease generally is dominated by the metastatic and/or local spread of the tumor. The aim of this paper is to deal with metastases from gastrointestinal cancer, particularly with pulmonary metastases, their incidence and their role within the pattern of metastases. Gastric cancer and colorectal cancer will be the main topics since they are the most common gastrointestinal malignancies. Surgery and chemotherapy as options for treatment of pulmonary lesions will be discussed briefly.

Pattern of Metastases

Autopsy data show very clearly that for all gastrointestinal tumors the liver is the key metastatic organ for blood-borne metastases [44]. Via liver the lungs may be involved next and from there distribution throughout the whole body may occur.

In table I the incidence of metastases from gastrointestinal malignancies is shown. These data are based on autopsied cases [48]. For all listed tumors the liver and the lungs are the most frequently involved organs. Lung metastases alone (multiple or solitary) occur only in a

Table I. Incidence of metastases from gastrointestinal tumors (from [49])

Primary tumor	Bone	Lung	Liver	Brain	Lung (only)
Esophagus	4– 7%	20–35%	20–32%	1%	17%
Stomach	5–10%	20–30%	35–50%	1–4%	7%
Pancreas	5–10%	25–40%	50–87%	1–4%	3%
Colon/rectum	5–10%	20–43%	71%	1%	9%

Table II. Pattern of lung and liver metastases from gastrointestinal tumors (modified from [45])

Primary tumor	– Lung – liver %	+ Lung + liver %	+ Lung – liver %	– Lung + liver %
Esophagus	60.0	16.6	16.6	6.6
Stomach	40.3	25.9	7.2	26.6
Pancreas	14.0	35.1	3.5	47.4
Colon	32.7	34.6	9.7	23.0
Rectum	38.9	31.5	12.1	17.5

minority of cases. Certain exemptions are the tumors of the esophagus and of the rectum. 17% of cases with esophageal cancer presented lung involvement only. Esophageal cancer can seed the lung in two ways: either directly by the azygos and semi-azygos veins or indirectly through the liver. Thus, in cancer of the esophagus, lungs and liver may play the part of the first filter for blood-borne metastases. The tumors of the rectum may drain along two vein systems. Via the middle hemorrhoidal veins directly to the lungs or via the superior hemorrhoidal vein system to the liver. Particularly tumors of the lower rectum are able to seed the lungs directly. The quoted 9% lung metastases only from colorectal cancer are certainly to a great extent due to malignancies of the lower rectum.

In table II the metastatic pattern concerning liver and lung involvement is listed more in detail. Again, these data are derived from autopsied cases [44]. Apart from esophageal cancer and rectal cancer, metastases to the liver alone are far more frequent than lung metastases alone. The high figures for no liver/no lung lesions reflect the local spread of the disease. Only occasionally are other organs seeded by metastases without prior liver and/or lung involvement. Of course this does not hold true for lymph node involvement. The occupation of the lymphatic system follows its own course of metastatic spread.

Other investigators [10] found a higher percentage of lung metastases alone from colorectal cancer than the data outlined above suggest, claiming also that a significant number of patients with upper rectal cancer presented lung metastases only. In these studies, however, the presence or absence of metastases was determined by clinical examination. Subclinical hepatic metastases may have remained undetected by these means. Since other authors [2, 15, 49] confirm the above-mentioned autopsy data, they must be considered to be more accurate than the results from clinical investigations. The fact that there is an obvious discrepancy between clinical data and autopsy data cannot be the crucial point for criticism [15]. The point is that clinical methods might lead to an overestimation of lung metastases (solely) from these tumors. In order to find out how close our own clinical staging procedures for patients treated within clinical trials come to the 'truth' presented by autopsy studies, we analyzed 88 patients with colorectal cancer (56 colon, 32 rectum) treated at the 'Onkologisches Zentrum, Mannheim' (Oncology Center, Mannheim) in phase-II trials between 1983 and 1986, and 77 patients with gastric cancer treated in clinical trials by the 'Chemotherapiegruppe Gastrointestinaler Tumoren' (Chemotherapy Group for Gastrointestinal Tumors) (CGT) from 1983 to 1986. The results are shown in table III. Only one patient with gastric carcinoma presented lung metastases alone. The majority of patients with gastric cancer had liver metastases (39%) and local recurrence or advanced

Table III. Pattern of lung and liver metastases from cancer of the stomach, colon, and rectum; clinical data of 88 patients with colorectal carcinoma (56 colon, 32 rectum) and 77 patients with gastric cancer. All patients were referred to the Onkologisches Zentrum Mannheim or hospitals of the Chemotherapiegruppe Gastrointestinaler Tumoren (CGT) during 1983 and 1986 and received chemotherapy within clinical trials

Primary tumor	− Lung − liver %	+ Lung + liver %	+ Lung − liver %	− Lung + liver %	Lung (only) %
Stomach	59.0	7.5	2.0	31.5	1.0
Colon	23.0	14.0	16.0	47.0	11.0
Rectum	15.5	34.5	25.0	25.0	16.0

local spread (59%). Only 12 of 77 patients (15.5%) had disease restricted to one site only.

In colorectal cancer a clearly higher percentage of patients was seen with tumor manifestation solely in one site (colon: 49%, rectum: 41%). Pulmonary metastases alone occurred in 11% of patients with colon tumors and in 16% of patients with cancer of the rectum. Combined metastases of liver and lung showed 14% of colon cancer patients but 34.5% of patients with carcinoma of the rectum. Liver metastases without pulmonary involvement were present in 47% of colon cancer patients and in 25% of patients with rectal carcinoma.

Although the numbers are very small, our clinical data are well in accordance with the autopsy studies cited above. About 10−15% of colorectal cancer patients can be expected to present clinically lung metastases only. This condition is more likely in patients with rectal cancer than in those with colon cancer. Few patients with gastric cancer will develop lung metastases only.

Prognostic Value of Lung Metastases

In 146 patients with advanced gastric carcinoma, survival and response to chemotherapy was related to localization of metastases [14]. All patients were treated in phase-III studies carried out by the CGT.

42% of patients had liver metastases, 34% lymph node involvement, 8% lung metastases, 9% metastatic occupation of the omentum, 34% peritoneal carcinosis and 58% local tumors (inoperable primary or local relapse).

Patients with pulmonary metastases showed a very poor prognosis (median survival time: 2.8 months) compared to those without lung involvement (median survival: 5.5 months). The same holds true for liver metastases: 3.4 months versus 5.6 months median survival time. Regarding response to chemotherapy, there was a tendency towards poor response in the group with liver metastases and there was no responder in the group with pulmonary metastases. For the latter the numbers of patients were too small to carry out correct statistical analysis. Other metastatic sites did not significantly influence survival and/or response to chemotherapy. Only patients with peritoneal metastases showed significantly higher response rates.

Concerning liver and lung metastases, these results confirm the data from other investigators [23, 29].

Lung metastases seem to be no special event in the course of gastric cancer. They more or less indicate the advanced stage of the disease. Therefore, the poor prognosis associated with lung involvement from gastric cancer is due to the disseminated stage of the malignancy and not to lung metastases themselves.

In 139 patients with colorectal cancer the prognostic value of metastatic sites for survival and response to chemotherapy was analysed [3]. All patients were treated in clinical trials in the Oncology Center in Mannheim.

28% of patients had liver metastases only, 30% liver and other sites, 12% other organs without liver, 8% lung metastases, 14% local recurrence or inoperable primary tumor, 6% intraabdominal lesions and 2% various other metastases.

Patients with local recurrence or inoperable primary tumor showed a significantly longer survival time than patients with multiple metastases and a slightly longer survival than patients with liver involvement. The shortest survival was observed in patients with multiple lesions without liver metastases (median survival: 4.5 months), the longest survival (10 months) in patients with local recurrence or inoperable primary tumor.

These results confirm two theses:

(1) Patients with local recurrence or inoperable primary tumor show a better prognosis than patients with distant metastases [30, 36, 38];

(2) patients with multiple lesions have the worst prognosis [18, 42].

A pronounced unfavourable influence of liver metastases as claimed by a number of authors [4, 21, 22] was not observed.

Response to chemotherapy was not influenced by number and localization of lesions.

A special role of lung metastases regarding survival and/or response to chemotherapy could not be identified. As in gastric cancer, lung metastases from colorectal cancer usually indicate a disseminated advanced stage of disease. An exemption are the few patients where lung involvement is the only manifestation of tumor.

Therapy of Lung Metastases

Two situations with existing lung metastases should be distinguished:
(1) Lung metastases as part of advanced disease with other organs

also involved. These patients will require systemic therapy. For recent updates on chemotherapy of gastric and colorectal cancer see [17] and [39].

(2) Pulmonary metastases alone without evident tumor manifestation elsewhere in the body. For this group of patients surgical removal of lesions might be a chance of cure.

Surgical excision of pulmonary metastases from colorectal cancer resulted in median survival times after thoracotomy of 27 months, ranging up to 42 months. Five-year survival rates were as high as 38% [5, 18, 25–27, 32–34, 41, 50]. Generally, patients with solitary lesions had a better prognosis than those with multiple metastases. These results are combined figures from rectal and colonic primary tumors. Separating the two groups, cancer of the rectum and cancer of the colon, there is no 5-year survival for patients with surgically removed lung metastases from colonic primary cancer but a 52% 5-year survival rate for patients with surgically removed lung metastases from rectal cancer [45].

These results illustrate very well the differences mentioned earlier in the pattern of metastases from colonic and rectal cancer.

Another aspect of solitary lung shadows in patients with a history of colonic cancer is described by a report from the Memorial Sloan-Kettering Cancer Center, New York [5]. Of 54 patients with known colon cancer who developed a metachronous or synchronous solitary lung shadow only 25 had metastases from colon cancer. Twenty-nine patients presented primary lung cancer.

Conclusions

For all gastrointestinal tract malignancies the key organ of blood-borne metastases is the liver. Usually occupation of the lungs is a second step in the metastatic process. For anatomical reasons esophageal and rectal cancer can have a different pattern of metastases. They are able to seed the lungs directly.

The incidence of lung metastases from gastrointestinal tract malignancies is 20–40%; the incidence of lung metastases alone (multiple or solitary) is 3–17%.

Pulmonary lesions from gastric and colorectal cancer do not particularly influence survival and/or response to chemotherapy.

Usually metastatic occupation of the lungs indicates advanced disseminated disease. In these conditions systemic treatment is required. A specific treatment for lung metastases is not available.

In cases of lung metastases alone (multiple or solitary) from gastrointestinal tumors surgery might be the treatment of choice. Particularly for solitary pulmonary lesions from rectal cancer the figures (5-year survival rate: 52%) suggest that surgery can offer a chance for cure to this small group of patients.

References

1   Bross, I. D. J.; Blumenson, L. E.: Metastatic sites that produce generalized cancer: Identification and kinetics of generalizing sites; in: Weiss, Fundamental aspects of metastatis, pp. 359–375 (Elsevier, New York 1976).

2   Brown, C. E.; Warren, S.: Visceral metastasis from rectal carcinoma. Surgery Gynec. Obstet. 66: 611–621 (1938).

3   Brummer, T.: Prognostische Faktoren des fortgeschrittenen kolorectalen Karzinoms unter Chemotherapie. Dissertation, Mannheim (1986).

4   Cady, B.; Oberfield, R. A.: Regional infusion chemotherapy of hepatic metastases from carcinoma of the colon. Am. J. Surg. 127: 220–227 (1974).

5   Cahan, W. G.; Castro, E. B.; Hajdu, S. I.: The significance of a solitary lung shadow in patients with colon carcinoma. Cancer 33: 414–421 (1974).

6   Chlebowski, R. T.; Silverberg, I.; Pajak, T. et al.: Treatment of advanced colon cancer with 5-fluorouracil (NSC 19893) versus cyclophosphamide (NSC 26271) plus 5-fluorouracil. Prognostic aspects of the differential white blood cell count. Cancer 45: 2240–2244 (1980).

7   Clarke, J. S.; Cruze, K.; El Farra, S.; Longmire, W. P., Jr.: The natural history and results of surgical therapy for carcinoma of the stomach. An analysis of 250 cases. Am. J. Surg. 102: 143 (1961).

8   Cohn, I., Jr.: The meaning of lymph node metastases and their treatment: Cancer of the stomach, pancreas, and small bowel; in: Weiss, Gilbert, Ballon, Lymphatic system metastases, pp. 262–274 (Hall, Boston 1980).

9   Cullinan, S. A.; Moertel, C. G.; Fleming, T. R.; Rubin, J. R.; Krook, J. E.; Everson, L. K.; Windschitl, H. E.; Twito, D. I.; Marschke, R. F.; Foley, J. F.; Pfeifle, D. M.; Barlow, J. F., for the North Central Cancer Treatment Group: A comparison of three chemotherapeutic regimens in the treatment of advanced pancreatic and gastric carcinoma. JAMA 253: 2061–2067 (1985).

10 Dionne, L.: The pattern of blood-borne metastasis from carcinoma of rectum. Cancer 18: 775–781 (1965).

11 Duarte, I.; Llanos, O.: Patterns of metastases in intestinal and diffuse types of carcinoma of the stomach. Human Pathol. 12: 237–242 (1981).

12 Dupont, J. B., Jr.; Cohn, I., Jr.: Gastric adenocarcinoma. Curr. Probl. Cancer 4: 25 (1980).

13 Dupont, J. B., Jr.; Lee, J. R.; Burton, G. R. et al.: Adenocarcinoma of the stomach: Review of 1497 cases. Cancer 41: 941 (1978).

14 Furkert, J.: Prognostische Faktoren beim chemotherapeutisch behandelten fortgeschrittenen Magenkarzinom. Dissertation, Mannheim (1985).

15 Gilbert, H. A.; Kagan, A. R.: Metastases: incidence, detection, and evaluation without histologic confirmation; in: Weiss, Fundamental aspects of metastasis, pp. 385–405 (Elsevier, New York 1976).

16 Godwin, J. D.; Brown, C. C.: Some prognostic factors in survival of patients with cancer of the colon and rectum. J. Chronic. Dis. *28:* 441–457 (1975).

17 Heim, M. E.; Worst, P.: Neuere Aspekte in der medikamentösen Therapie fortgeschrittener kolorektaler Karzinome. Akt. Onkologie, vol. 33, pp. 102–124 (Zuckschwerdt, München 1986).

18 Hughes, E. S.; McConchie, I. H.; McDermott, F. T. et al.: Resection of lung metastases in large bowel cancer. Br. J. Surg. *69:* 410–412 (1982).

19 Kayser, K.; Burkhardt, H.-U.: The incidence of gastrointestinal cancer in North-Baden (West Germany) 1971–1977. J. Cancer Res. clin. Oncol. *93:* 301–321 (1979).

20 Kemeny, N.; Braun, D. W.: Prognostic factors in advanced colorectal carcinoma. Am. J. Med. *74:* 786–794 (1983).

21 Kemeny, N.; Yagoda, A.; Braun, D.: Metastatic colorectal carcinoma. A prospective randomised trial of methyl-CCNU, 5-fluorouracil (5-FU) and vincristine (MOF) versus MOF plus streptozotocin (MOF-strep). Cancer *51:* 20–24 (1983).

22 Lavin, P. T.; Mittelman, A.; Douglass, H. et al.: Survival and response to chemotherapy for advanced colorectal adenocarcinoma. An Eastern Cooperative Oncology Group report. Cancer *46:* 1536–1543 (1980).

23 Lavin, P. T.; Bruckner, H. W.; Plaxe, S. C.: Studies in prognostic factors relating to chemotherapy for advanced gastric cancer. Cancer *50:* 2016–2023 (1982).

24 MacDonald, J. S.; Schein, P. S.; Woolley, P. V. et al.: 5-fluorouracil, doxorubicin, and mitomycin C (FAM) combination chemotherapy for advanced gastric cancer. Ann. intern. Med. *93:* 533–536 (1980).

25 Mansel, J. K.; Zinsmeister, A. R.; Pairolero, P. C.; Jett, J. R.: Pulmonary resection of metastatic colorectal adenocarcinoma. A ten year experience. Chest *89:* 109 (1986).

26 McCormack, P. M.; Attiyeh, F. F.: Resected pulmonary metastases from colorectal cancer. Dis. Colon Rectum *22:* 553–556 (1979).

27 McCormack, P. M.; Bains, M. S.; Beattie, E. J., Jr.; Martini, N.: Pulmonary resection in metastatic carcinoma. Chest *73:* 163–166 (1978).

28 Moertel, C. G.: The natural history of advanced gastric cancer. Surg. Gynec. Obstet. *128:* 1071–1074 (1968).

29 Moertel, C. G.: Carcinoma of the stomach: Prognostic factors and criteria of response to therapy; in: Staquet, Cancer therapy: Prognostic factors and criteria of response, pp. 229–236 (Raven Press, New York 1975).

30 Moertel, C. G.; Reitemeier, R. L.: Advanced gastrointestinal cancer. Clinical management and chemotherapy (Harper & Row, New York, London 1969).

31 Moertel, C. G.; Mittelman, J. A.; Bakemeier, R. F. et al.: Sequential and combination chemotherapy of advanced cancer. Cancer *38:* 678–682 (1976).

32 Morrow, C. E.; Vassilopoulos, P.; Grage, T. B.: Surgical resection for metastatic neoplasms of the lung. Cancer *45:* 2981–2985 (1981).

33 Mountain, C. F.; McMurtrey, M. J.: Surgery for pulmonary metastasis: a 20-year experience. 20th Anniversary Meeting of the Society of Thoracic Surgeons, San Antonio, Tx. 1984.

34 Mountain, C. F.; Khalil, K. G.; Hermes, K. E. et al.: The contributions of surgery to the management of carcinomatous pulmonary metastases. Cancer *41*: 833–840 (1978).

35 Papachristou, D. N.; Fortner, J. G.: Local recurrence of gastric adenocarcinomas after gastrectomy. J. surg. Oncol. *18*: 47–53 (1981).

36 Pestana, C.; Reitemeier, R. J.; Moertel, C. G. et al.: The natural history of carcinoma of the colon and rectum. Am. J. Surg. *108*: 826–829 (1964).

37 Pickren, J. W.: Use and limitations of autopsy data; in: Weiss, Fundamental aspects of metastasis, pp. 377–381 (Elsevier, New York 1976).

38 Pihl, E.; Hughes, E. S. R.; McDermott, F. T. et al.: Carcinoma of the rectum and rectosigmoid: cancer specific long term survival. Cancer *45*: 2902–2907 (1980).

39 Queißer, W.; Flechtner, H.: Chemotherapy of advanced gastric carcinoma. Onkologie *9*: 319–331 (1986).

40 Richards, F.; Pajak, T. L.; Cooper, M. R.; Spurr, C. L.: Comparison of 5-fluorouracil, cyclophosphamide, and methotrexate in metastatic colorectal carcinoma. Cancer *36*: 1589–1592 (1975).

41 Schulten, M. F.; Heiskell, C. A.; Shields, T. W.: The incidence of solitary pulmonary metastasis from carcinoma of the large intestine. Surg. Gynec. Obstet. *143*: 727–729 (1976).

42 Silverman, D. T.; Murray, J. L.; Smart, C. R. et al.: Estimated median survival times of patients with colorectal cancer based on experience with 9745 patients. Am. J. Surg. *133*: 289–297 (1977).

43 Statistisches Jahrbuch 1985 für die Bundesrepublik Deutschland. (Statistisches Bundesamt, Wiesbaden 1986).

44 Viadana, E.; Bross, I. D.; Pickren, J. W.: Cascade spread of blood-borne metastases in solid and nonsolid cancers of humans; in: Weiss, Gilbert, Pulmonary metastasis, pp. 143–167 (Hall, Boston 1978).

45 Vincent, R. G.; Choksi, L. B.; Takita, H. et al.: Surgical resection of the solitary pulmonary metastasis; in: Weiss, Gilbert, Pulmonary metastasis, pp. 232–242 (Hall, Boston 1978).

46 Warren, S.: Studies on tumor metastases: IV. Metastases of cancer of the stomach. New Engl. J. Med. *209*: 825 (1933).

47 Warwick, M.: Analysis of one hundred and seventy-six cases of carcinoma of the stomach submitted to autopsy. Ann. Surg. *88*: 216 (1928).

48 Weiss, L.; Gilbert, H. A.: Introduction; in: Weiss, Gilbert, Pulmonary metastasis, pp. 100–103 (Hall, Boston, 1978).

49 Willis, R. A.: The spread of tumors in the human body (Butterworth, London 1973).

50 Wilking, N.; Petrelli, N. J.; Herrera, L. et al.: Surgical resection of pulmonary metastases from colorectal adenocarcinoma. Dis. Colon Rectum *28*: 562–564 (1985).

Dr. med. H. Flechtner, Onkologisches Zentrum, Klinikum Mannheim,
Fakultät für klinische Medizin der Universität Heidelberg,
Theodor-Kutzer-Ufer, D-6800 Mannheim (FRG)

Contr. Oncol., vol. 30, pp. 195–207 (Karger, Basel 1988)

Renal Cell Carcinoma

K. Possinger[a, b], H. Wagner[a], R. Beck[a], A. Staebler[a], L. Schmid[c], B. Vollmann[c], W. Wilmanns[a, b]

[a] Medizinische Klinik III der Universität München, Klinikum Großhadern, München, FRG
[b] Gesellschaft für Strahlen- und Umweltforschung, München Neuherberg, FRG
[c] Onkologische Klinik Oberstaufen; Oberstaufen, FRG

Introduction

Malignant neoplasma of the kidney belongs to the rarer forms of cancer. The highest mortality rate for kidney tumors is found in Northern Europe, the lowest in Southern and Eastern Europe. In the Federal Republic of Germany the incidence is 7.7 for men and 3.5 for women per 100,000 population per year [23]. During the last few years, the mortality has shown a slight increase. To find parameters related to the prognosis of renal cell carcinoma, we analyzed 97 patients with this tumor, seen between 1981 and 1986 in our hospital in Großhadern.

The so-called 'classic triad' of hematuria, flank pain and abdominal mass was present in only 5% of our patients. The most common symptom was gross hematuria [1]. In more than one-third of our patients, distant metastases led to the detection of the primary tumor.

Whereas the natural history of renal cell carcinoma may vary extremely from person to person, the one-year survival rate, calculated from the manifestation of distant metastases, is less than 20% [2,3]. This extremely rapid tumor progression after the manifestation of the metastases is in striking contradiction to the opinion, even stated by oncologists, that advanced renal cell carcinoma is a relatively slowly progressing tumor! This false conclusion probably depends on the fact that patients with these carcinomas rarely undergo routine controls in large numbers. It is true that the renal cell carcinoma has the second highest reported incidence of spontaneous regression, surpassed only by melanoma, but the incidence of this regression is less than 1%. Up to now, approximately 70 cases of spontaneous regression of renal cell carcinoma have been reported in the literature [4, 5]. In an excellent review, DeKernion and Berry [5] analyzed the incidence of such tumor regressions and their clinical or autopsy validation: out of more than 1,000 patients with renal cell carcinoma, they detected only 5 persons with tumor regression (0.4%!). In addition to this, the authors pointed out that the opinion that a nephrectomy would promote spontaneous remission of metastases represents much more a wish than a clinical reality (table I, II). Among our patients, there was not one case of a spontaneous tumor remission; in addition to this, we did not find any nephrectomy-induced remission of tumor metastases. In some patients, we got confirmation of the well-known phenomenon that metastatic foci stop growing for a long time, and then are followed by a sudden increase in size.

More than half of our patients had distant metastases either at the time of diagnosis of the primary tumor or developed them during the first postoperative year. The main metastatic sites were the skeletal system, the lymph nodes and the liver.

Table I. Frequency of spontaneous tumor remissions in patients with renal cell carcinoma

Author*	Year	No. of patients	Spontaneous remissions
Riches	1964	130	0
Mims	1966	97	1
V. Schreeb	1967	232	0
Middleton	1967	100	0
Markewitz	1967	141	0
Rafla	1970	244	0
Skinner	1972	77	1
Bloom	1973	195	2
Montie	1977	78	0
DeKernion	1978	86	1
Possinger	1986	97	0
Total		1,447	5 (0.345%)

* Complete references available from authors on request.

Table II. Spontaneous remissions of tumor metastases after nephrectomy

Author*	Year	No. of patients	Spontaneous remissions
Mims	1966	57	1
Middleton	1967	33	0
Myers	1968	20	0
Rafla	1970	14	0
Bottiger	1970	100	0
Wagle	1970	80	2
Skinner	1972	77	1
Johnson	1975	43	0
Lokich	1975	45	0
Montie	1977	25	0
Patel	1978	25	0
DeKernion	1978	52	0
Possinger	1986	92	0

* Complete references available from authors on request.

Prognostic Factors

With the aid of specific prognostic factors, it seems to be possible to estimate the individual course of the disease already at the time of the first diagnosis of the tumor. Similar to patients with breast cancer, the probability of survival correlates much more with the stage of the disease (regional lymph node infiltration, infiltration of the surrounding organs) than with the size of the primary tumor. The invasion of the tumor in the Vena renalis does not have an unfavorable impact on the course of the disease. On the other hand, the histological grading is an important prognostic factor in that well-differentiated tumors have a better prognosis than poorly-differentiated tumors [6]. We examined the influence on survival of age, sex, duration of disease-free interval, metastatic site and the number of infiltrated organs. Similarly, we screened the hematocrit levels and the erythrocyte sedimentation rate as prognostic parameters.

The statistical analysis of the data was performed by the Kaplan-Meier product limit estimation and by specific types of the log rank test [7−12].

Age

The median age at diagnosis was 55 years (lower quartile < 49, upper quartile > 62 years). In order to evaluate the influence of age on the course of the disease, we compared the survival of patients younger than 49 years with those aged between 49 and 61 and over 61 years. The median survival of the patients younger than 49 years and older than 61 years was 22 months and 18 months, respectively, whereas the group in the middle survived for 36 months. This difference does not include a statistical significance. Analyzed from the first appearance of distant metastases, there was only a minor difference in survival time between the 3 groups (fig. 1, 2). Based on these data, we believe that, similar to most other solid tumors, age does not have a significant influence on the further course of the disease. The same holds true for patients suffering from renal cell carcinoma [13].

Sex

As most of the spontaneous tumor remissions are to be found in male patients, and as in addition to this, in experiments with animals, the incidence as well as the growth of estrogen-induced renal cell carci-

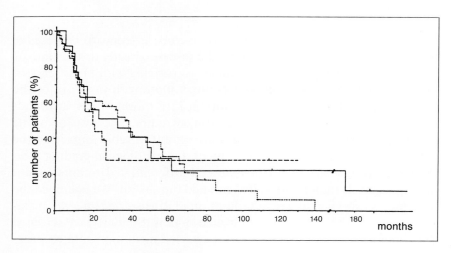

Fig. 1. Cumulative survival (%) of 97 patients with metastasized renal cell carcinoma, depending on age, calculated from the time of the first diagnosis.
≤ 48 years: ——, n = 26; 49–61 years: ······, n = 44; ≥ 62 years: – – –, n = 27; p = no statistical significance.

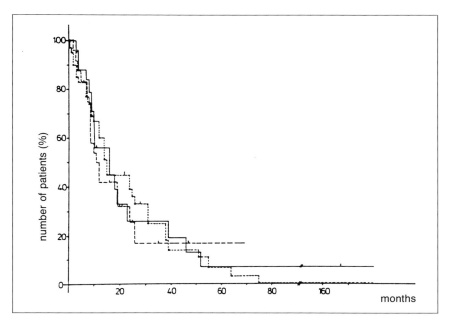

Fig. 2. Cumulative survival (%) depending on age, calculated from the first occur-rance of metastases. ≤ 48 years: ———, n = 25; 49–61 years: ······, n = 40; ≥ 62 years: − − −, n = 24; p = no statistical significance.

nomas are suppressed by testosterone, we examined how far sex is re-sponsible for a different course of the disease. We found out that the median survival times of the 61 male and 36 female patients, which were 22 and 26.5 months respectively, calculated from the time of the first diagnosis, and 14 and 10 months respectively, from the first occurrence of distant metastases, showed only a minor difference (fig. 3). The fact that renal cell carcinoma occurs in male patients almost twice as often as in female patients shows that the dependence upon hormones in ex-periments with animals does not have any relevance for humans.

Disease Free Interval

De Kernion et al. [14] stressed in their publications the prognostic value of the disease-free interval. They found out that patients with a long disease-free interval (> 24 months) had survived considerably

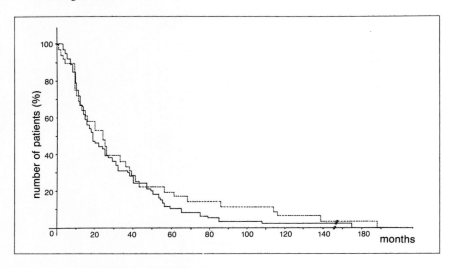

Fig. 3. Cumulative survival (%) depending on sex, calculated from the time of the first diagnosis. Male: ———, n = 61; female: – – –, n = 36; p = no statistical signif-icance.

longer than patients with a short disease-free interval ($<$ 6 months). We could state the same significant difference ($p < 0.001$) with our pa-tients. Nevertheless, from the time of the occurrence of distant metasta-ses onward, patients with a long disease-free interval could no longer enjoy an advantage in their survival time (fig. 4)! The median survival time (11.5 and 14.5 months respectively) was not significantly different!

Number of Infiltrated Organs and Tumor Sites
The extent of the metastatic sites and especially the localization of the tumors seem to be of considerable importance for the remaining survival time: Patients with only one infiltrated organ survived more than twice as long as patients with two or more carcinomatous, infil-trated organs (18.5 versus 8.5 months, see fig. 5)!

Patients with metastases in the skeletal system or the soft tissue sur-vived significantly longer than patients with metastases in the lungs or the liver ($p = 0.02$): The median time of survival for patients with bone metastases was 33 months, with infiltration in the lungs, 12 months, and with liver metastases only 10.5 months (fig. 6).

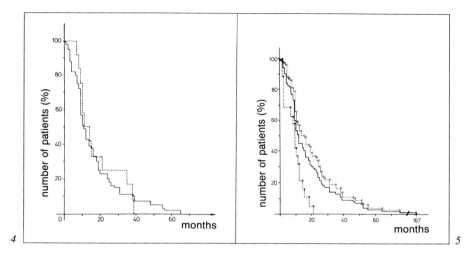

Fig. 4. Cumulative survival (%) depending on the disease-free interval, calculated from the first occurrence of metastases. Short interval: ≤ 6 months: ———, n = 61; long interval: ≥ 24 months: – – –, n = 12; p = no statistical significance.

Fig. 5. Cumulative survival (%) of 97 patients (total: ———) depending on the number of the carcinomatous, infiltrated organs, calculated from the first occurrence of metastases. 1 organ: ○ ○ ○, n = 70; 2 or more organs: ● ● ●, n = 27; p = 0.0008.

Hematocrit and Erythrocyte Sedimentation Rate

According to publications by Smith, Riches and Sufrin [15, 16] an increased level of erythropoietin concomitant with a reactive polyglobulia should be considered a favorable prognostic parameter. Therefore, we examined in our patients how far increased levels of hematocrit (46%) and decreased erythrocyte sedimentation rates (5 mm: 1 h, Westergreen), measured at the time of the tumor diagnosis, correlated with the course of the disease. In agreement with the results of Smith et al. [15], we found that patients with elevated hematocrit levels survived significantly longer than patients with normal or reduced levels (33 versus 18 months, see fig. 7). The erythrocyte sedimentation rate did not have a predictive value for the further course of the disease.

Hormonal and Cytotoxic Therapy

Whether systemic treatment modalities with hormones or cytotoxic drugs have an influence on the survival time remains controversial. In-

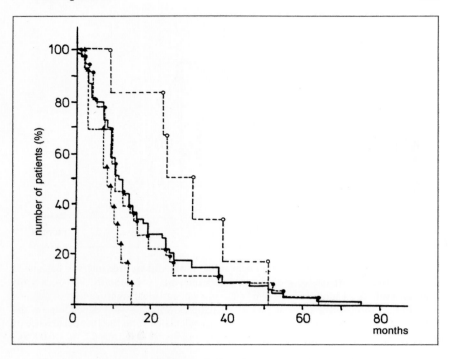

Fig. 6. Cumulative survival (%) of 97 patients (total: ———) with primary metastases in the bones: ○ ○ ○, n = 6; in the lungs: ● ● ●, n = 36; and in the liver: ▲▲▲,
n = 13; calculated from the first occurrence of metastases. (o.v. ●: p = 0.02).

deed, in a clinical trial by the Eastern Cooperative Oncology Group
(ECOG) [17] it was pointed out that patients showing a tumor remission
during anti-estrogen therapy survive significantly longer than patients
with tumor progression; however, it was not explained in this publication whether this effect was really induced by the therapy, or if this
advantage was hypothesized in 2 groups of patients with different prognostic criteria! We examined, in 67 patients, the impact of systemic
therapy (Tamoxifen®, medac, Hamburg, FRG: 40 mg/day, p.o., and
vinblastine: 3−5 mg/week, i.v.) on the survival time. We selected these
drugs because of their low systemic toxicity and their − at least as
reported in the literature [17−19] − limited efficacy. Entry criteria for
the study were the occurrence of visceral metastases and documented

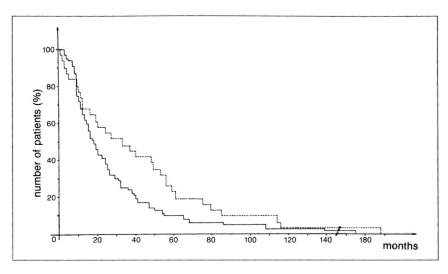

Fig. 7. Cumulative survival (%) depending on hematocrit, calculated from the time of the first diagnosis. Low hematocrit ≤ 41: – – –, n = 31; high hematocrit ≥ 46: ———, n = 63; (p = 0.05).

progressive disease. While following the combination therapy, 10 patients achieved an objective tumor remission, and 24 patients a disease stabilization for at least 3 months. The other patients experienced tumor progression in spite of systemic treatment [20]. The therapeutic response was classified according to the WHO criteria [21].

Comparing the survival time of the patients with objective remission and patients with progressive disease, a striking difference could be demonstrated (p = 0.0002, see fig. 8), but a detailed subgrouping of our patients according to prognostic factors demonstrated that the majority of the patients with tumor progression had unfavorable prognostic criteria and that patients with stable disease or objective remission showed a predominance of favorable prognostic factors. Upon evaluating the impact of the systemic therapy on the survival time of the patients, separated into groups with favorable and unfavorable prognostic criteria, we did not find any difference! This seems to us to be a strong indication that systemic treatment has no influence on the survival time.

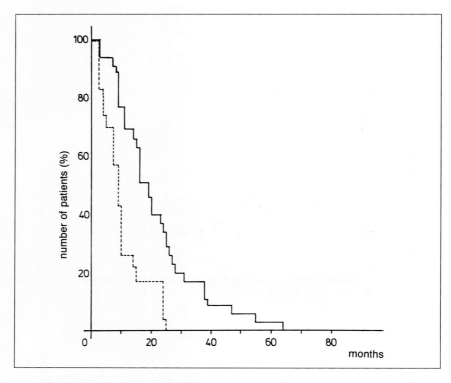

Fig. 8. Cumulative survival (%) depending on the response to systemic chemotherapy, calculated from the first occurrence of metastases: a seemingly therapeutically
induced advantage of survival (p = 0.0002) is in reality caused by the selection of 2 patient subgroups with different prognostic factors: objective remission + stable disease:
———, n = 35; progressive disease: – – –, n = 20.

Excision of Metastases

To alter the fateful course of the disease in patients with metastasized renal cell carcinoma, surgical excision of metastases was performed
in some patients, if they had regionally limited or solitary metastases.
But because of the small number of patients, the statistical analysis has
failed up to now to demonstrate a significant improvement of survival,
induced by the excision of the metastases. DeKernion et al. reported the
course of disease in 20 patients with surgical resection of tumor metastases. The authors referred to the remarkably long survival times in

these patients [14]. In 20 of our patients, surgical excisions of metastases were also performed. In 6 of these patients, solitary or regionally limited pulmonary metastases were excised; in the other 14 patients, skeletal and/or soft tissue metastases were removed. Though the median survival of the surgically treated patients was remarkably longer (21 versus 13 months) compared with the other patients, no significant difference in survival could be demonstrated (p = 0.8, see fig. 9).

Since, on the one hand, we do not have a really effective treatment modality for patients with metastasized renal cell carcinoma at present, and since, on the other hand, the surgical excision of tumor metastases results in only limited morbidity in the patient, this approach should be taken into account in each patient with solitary or regionally limited metastases.

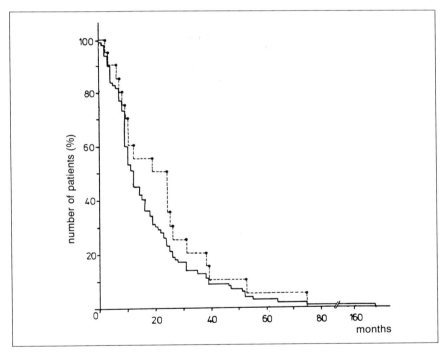

Fig. 9. Cumulative survival (%) of 97 patients with and without excision of metastases, calculated from the first occurrence of metastases. No excision: ———, n = 77; excision: – – –, n = 20; (p = 0.8).

References

1   Possinger, K.; Hartenstein, R.; Erhart, H.: Klinik und Chemotherapie des Adeno-karzinoms der Niere. Fortschr. Med. *99:* 419–424 (1981).

2   Hindmarsh, J. R.; Hall, R. R.; Kulatilake, A. E.: Renal cell carcinoma. A prelimi-nary clinical trial of methodichlorophen (D.D.M.P.) Clin. Oncol. *5:* 11 (1979).

3   Kats, S. A.; Davis, J. E.: Renal Adenocarcinoma. Prognosis and treatment reflected by survival. Urology *10:* 10–11 (1977).

4   Freed, S. Z.; Halpirin, J. P.; Gordon, M.: Idiopathic regression of metastases from renal cell carcinoma. J. Urol. *118:* 538–542 (1977).

5   DeKernion, J. B.; Berry, D.: The diagnosis and treatment of renal cell carcinoma. Cancer *45:* 1947–1956 (1980).

6   Skinner, D. G.; Colvin, R. B.; Vermillion, C. D. et al.: Diagnosis and management of renal cell carcinoma. A clinical and pathologic study of 309 cases. Cancer *28:* 1165–1177 (1971).

7   Gehan, E. A.: A generalized Wilcoxon test for comparing arbitrarily singly cen-sored samples. Biometrika *52:* 203–223 (1965).

8   Peto, R.; Peto, J.: Asymptotically efficient rank invariant test procedures. J. R. Stat. Soc. Ass. *135:* 185–206 (1972).

9   Peto, R.; Pike, M. C.: Conservatism of the approximation $(0-E)^2/E$ in the logrank test for survival data or tumor incidence data. Biometrics *29:* 579–584 (1973).

10   Peto, R.; Pike, M. C. et al.: Design and analysis of randomised clinical trials requir-ing prolonged observation of each patient. I. Introduction and design. Br. J. Cancer *34:* 585–612 (1976).

11   Peto, R.; Pike, M. C. et al.: Design and analysis of randomised clinical trials requir-ing prolonged observation of each patient. II. Analysis and examples. Br. J. Cancer *35:* 1–37 (1977).

12   Rahlfs, V. W.; Wardenburg, H. von: Die Analyse zensierter Daten in der klinischen und pharmakologischen Forschung. Krebsgeschehen *15:* 117–126 (1983).

13   Wilmanns, W.; Biensack, T.; Sauer, H.: Zytostatische Polychemotherapie im höhe-ren Lebensalter. Dt. med. Wschr. *110:* 1959–1962 (1985).

14   DeKernion, J. B.; Ramming, K. P.; Smith, R. B.: The natural history of metastatic renal cell carcinoma: A computer analysis. J. Urol. *120:* 148–152 (1978).

15   Smith, H.; Riches, E.: Hemoglobin values in renal cell carcinoma. Lancet *i:* 1058 (1960).

16   Sufrin, G.; Mirand, E. A.; Moore, R. H. et al.: Hormons in renal cancer. J. Urol. *117:* 433 (1977).

17   Al-Sarraf, M.; Eyre, H.; Bonnet, J. et al.: Study of tamoxifen in metastatic renal cell carcinoma and the influence of certain prognostic factors: A south-west onco-logy group study. Cancer Treat. Rep. *65:* 447–451 (1981).

18   Bodey, G. P.: Current status of chemotherapy in metastatic renal cell carcinoma; in Johnson, Samuels, Cancer of the genito-urinary tract, pp. 67–72 (Raven, New York 1979).

19   DeKernion, J. B.; Berry, D.: The diagnosis and treatment of renal cell carcinoma. Cancer *45:* 1947–1986 (1980).

20   Wagner, H.; Possinger, K.; Wilmanns, W.: Therapie des metastasierenden Nieren-

zellkarzinoms. Phase-II-Studie: Kombinationstherapie Vinblastin/Tamoxifen. Z. analyt. Chem. *2:* 5–13 (1984).

21 WHO handbook for reporting results of cancer treatment (WHO Offset Publication 48, Geneva 1979).

22 McCormack, P.M.; Martini, N.: The changing role of surgery for pulmonary metastases. Ann. thor. Surg. *28:* 139–145 (1979).

23 Becker, N.; Frentzel-Beyme, R.; Wagner, G.: Atlas of cancer mortality in the Federal Republic of Germany (Springer, Berlin, Heidelberg, New York, Tokyo 1984).

Dr. med. K. Possinger, Medizinische Klinik III der Universität München, Klinikum Großhadern, Marchioninistraße 15, D-8000 München 70 (FRG)

Contr. Oncol., vol. 30, pp. 208–215 (Karger, Basel 1988)

Pulmonary Metastases in Malignant Melanoma

S. Ritter, H. Drepper

Fachklinik Hornheide, Münster, FRG

The material for this paper was collected in the TNM Field Study 'Malignant Melanoma' conducted at the 'Fachklinik Hornheide/ Münster' and supported by the Federal Government of the FRG. Reporting on behalf of this study group is Dr. Drepper. In the recruitment phase – March 6, 1980 to December 31, 1983 – 872 melanoma patients were entered into the study; follow-up was continued hereafter and continually documented.

Distant metastases were detected in one patient at first presentation, in 150 in the follow-up; 61 of these patients were found to have pulmonary metastases.

If a malignant melanoma develops hematogenous metastases, practically every organ may be involved. Pulmonary metastases are rather frequently the first distant manifestations. This may be partly due to their ready recognition by diagnostic radiology, but the metastatic pathways via lymph nodes into the venous circulation may also play an important role. In 27 patients, pulmonary foci were the first distant metastases observed; in 17 there were simultaneous other distant metastases. In 17 other patients, various other distant metastases had preceded the pulmonary manifestations.

The age distribution (table I) of the entire study group does not differ significantly from that of the subgroup with pulmonary metastases, but sex distribution shows a different pattern (table II). While women predominate in the entire group, the subgroup of patients with pulmonary metastases has a predominance of men, which correlates with the well-known poorer prognosis of male melanoma patients in general. The supposition that the prognosis of malignant melanoma depends

Table I. Age distribution

Age (years)	Entire study group (n = 872)	Patients with lung metastases (n = 61)
Under 20	8 (0.9%)	0
21–40	145 (16.6%)	15 (24.6%)
41–60	355 (40.7%)	20 (32.8%)
61–80	329 (37.8%)	25 (41.0%)
Over 80	35 (4.0%)	1 (1.6%)

Table II. Sex distribution

	n	Males	Females
Entire study group	872	343 (39.3%)	529 (60.7%)
Patients with lung metastases	61	37 (60.7%)	23 (39.3%)

Difference significant on the 1% level (χ^2-test)

Table III. In-depth level of the primary

	I + II*	II – III*	III*	III – IV*	IV*	V*
Entire study group (n = 809)	151 (18.7%)	8 (0.1%)	310 (38.3%)	3 (0.4%)	302 (37.3%)	35 (4.3%)
Patients with lung metastases (n = 56)	—	1 (1.8%)	14 (25.0%)	—	37 (66.1%)	4 (7.4%)

* Difference significant on the 1% level (χ^2-test)

mainly on the thickness of the primary tumor was confirmed by our data. Figure 1 shows that pulmonary metastases developed more often in patients with primary tumors larger than 3 mm than in the entire study group. The depth of invasion of the primary (table III) shows a similar, though less marked difference. Levels IV and V are represented

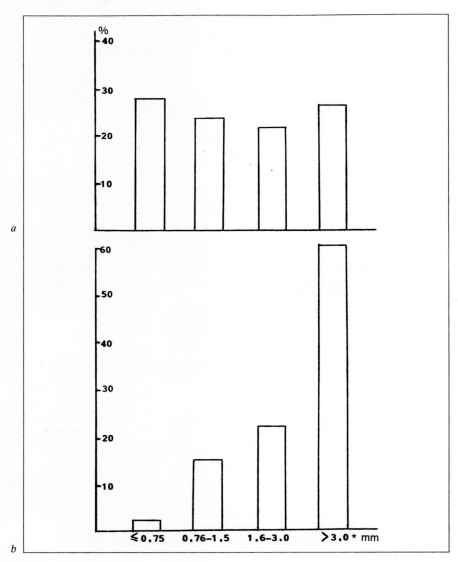

Fig. 1. Thickness of primary. *a* Entire collective, melanoma study (n = 809); *b* with lung metastases (n = 59). * = difference significant on the 1% level (χ^2-test).

in the pulmonary metastases group more often than in the total group. Thickness of the primary and depth of invasion are criteria of the T-stage (table IV). T_4 tumors are markedly more frequent among the patients with pulmonary metastases than among the entire group. With regard to staging which reflects the spread to surrounding tissues and regional lymph nodes, some difference is noted in stage II: Approximately 26% of patients with pulmonary metastases are found in this stage in contrast to 12% in the whole study collective (table V). The actual localization of the primary tumor (table VI) has no significant influence. The fact that the whole study group shows a somewhat higher percentage of localizations at the lower extremities seems to correlate with the divergent sex ratios: melanomas in women are frequently localized at a lower extremity.

Table IV. Postoperative T staging

	%				
	T_x	T_1*	T_2*	T_3	T_4*
Entire study group (n = 820)**	1.5	17.0	27.7	27.2	26.6
Patients with lung metastases (n = 60)	1.7	—	10.0	26.7	61.7

  * Difference significant on the 1% level (χ^2-test)
 ** except T_0, T_{is}

Table V. Postoperative staging (clinical)

	No data	I*	II*	IV
Entire study group (n = 857)	1 (0.1%)	749 (87.4%)	106 (12.4%)	1 (0.1%)
Patients with lung metastases (n = 61)	1 (1.6%)	43 (70.5%)	16 (26.2%)	1 (1.6%)

* Difference significant on the 1% level (χ_2-test)

Table VI. Localization of the primary (Fachklinik Hornheide, April 1986)

	Head and neck	Trunk	Upper extremities	Lower extremities	Genitals female/male	
Entire study group (n = 865)	225 (26.0%)	211 (24.4%)	149 (17.2%)	273 (31.6%)	6 (0.8%)	1
Patients with lung metastases (n = 61)	18 (29.5%)	15 (24.6%)	14 (22.9%)	12 (19.7%)	— (3.3%)	2

Table VII. Occurrence of lung metastases in 61 melanoma patients

After surgical removal of primary	As first distant metastases	Other distant metastases simultaneously	Other distant metastases previously	Total
Simultaneously	1	—	—	1
In the 1st year	4	4	—	8
2nd year	7	6	8	21
3rd year	8	4	6	18
4th year	4	2	3	9
5th year	3	1	—	4

Some aspects of the interval between surgical resection of the primary and the first manifestation of metastasis are shown in table VII. Only one patient had pulmonary metastases when the primary was operated. In general, metastasization manifested itself mostly 2 or 3 years after surgery; pulmonary metastases were detected during this period in 39 out of 61 patients.

What is the exact localization of such pulmonary metastases at the time of detection? The evaluation of 53 patients (table VIII) shows a relatively high proportion of initially solitary foci in the lung. This was the case in 25 patients. Eight patients had 2, and 20 had more than 2 metastases when they were discovered. In a number of patients additional pulmonary metastases developed rapidly.

Table IX shows the survival times after the manifestation of pulmonary metastases. Apparently it is less important whether they arise in

Table VIII. First manifestation of pulmonary metastases in 53 patients

	Right	Left	Bilateral	Total
Solitary	10	15	—	25 patients
2 metastases	6	1	1	8 patients
More than 2 metastases	5	2	13	20 patients

Table IX. Survival after the detection of lung metastases either solitary, or together with other distant metastases

Detection	n	Survival in months		Now living	
		from/to	mean	n	months
In the 1st year	7	1−12	7.0	1	35
2nd year	13	2−21	10.5	2	13, 16
3rd year	11	3−21	10.4	2	2+, ?
4th year	6	2−14	7.1	3	9, 6, 5
5th year	4	−	1.0	3	20, 14, ?
Total			9.1		

the first, second or third year after surgery; the mean survival time after metastasization was 9.1 months, with rather a wide range of deviations. However, the overall survival of a melanoma patient will depend essentially on the early or later occurrence of distant metastases. It should be emphasized that melanoma patients will rarely die of their pulmonary metastases, but rather of subsequent distant metastases, especially to the brain. Nearly all the patients in our study who died during the past few years succumbed to brain metastases, some to liver metastases.

The one patient in table IX has survived now for 35 months; he had a complete remission with regression of a pulmonary metastasis after chemotherapy.

Table X shows that survival after the occurrence of nonpulmonary distant metastases (17 patients with involvement of other organs) with a mean rate of 10.4 months, was not much different. In these patients,

Table X. Survival after detection of other distant metastases with subsequent pulmonary metastases

n	Survival in months				Living	
	other metastases		lung metastases			
	mean	range	mean	range	n	months
17	10.4	3 – 23	4.3	1 – 17	1	14.3

Table XI. Malignant melanoma. Distant metastases found in 74 autopsies (from [1])

Lung	76%
Liver	54%
Adrenal	51%
Brain	40%
Heart	40%
Kidney	38%
Bone	35%
Small intestine	34%
Pancreas	32%
Spleen	27%
Stomach	26%

Other organs from 1% (eyes)
to 24% (colon)

metastasization to the lung was noted somewhat later, and they did not survive for more than a few months.

Table XI summarizes an impressive autopsy statistic published by Meyer [1] with pulmonary involvement in 76%, and brain metastases in 40% of patients. Another remarkable fact is the frequency of cardiac metastases which may also often be the immediate cause of death. In 15 of our 61 patients with pulmonary metastases, brain involvement could be confirmed at autopsy.

Since they are rather readily recognized, metastases to the lung, like those to skin and lymph nodes, are taken as an important indicator of incipient distant metastasization. In high-risk melanomas, especially T_4 tumors and those at stage II (T_3, T_4, N_1), chest X-ray check-ups at regular intervals are particularly indicated. The data presented above will also stress the importance of early diagnosis.

Our own diagnostic procedure is focused on the greatest possible accuracy in assessing the extent of distant spread. Careful clinical examination is obligatory. X-ray diagnostics include thorax and, if suspicious, skeletal parts. CT examinations check the possible spread to the abdomen and brain. Bone metastases are traced by whole-body skeletal scintigraphy. Some laboratory parameters are also routinely controlled, although they are not very helpful for the detection of incipient metastases. All this information is pooled for the planning of therapy. In cases of solitary metastases to the lung, without distant involvement of other organs, surgical resection is indicated. If resective therapy is no longer possible − sometimes even in the case of cutaneous metastasization − chemotherapy is the next step; we prefer a combination of BCNU, hydroxyurea, and dacarbazine. Complete remissions have been achieved in several cases of pulmonary metastases, lasting for many months in some cases, even as long as 35 months in one patient who is still living.

Reference

1   Meyer, J. E.: Radiographic evaluation of metastatic melanoma. Cancer *42:* 127−132 (1978).

PD Dr. S. Ritter, Fachklinik Hornheide, Dorbaumstraße 300, D-4400 Münster (FRG)

Contr. Oncol., vol. 30, pp. 216–221 (Karger, Basel 1988)

Aspects of Surgery for Pulmonary Metastases in Soft Tissue Sarcoma in Adults

P. Schlag

Section of Surgical Oncology, Department of Surgery, University of Heidelberg, FRG

In 50–80% of the patients with high-grade sarcoma, metastases of the lung have to be expected. Metastases of the lung is the most frequent cause of mortality in soft tissue sarcoma. In over half the cases the lung is the first and only locality of metastases. Even in autopsy statistics it is shown that metastasizing is confined to the lung [5, 16].

The median survival time of patients without therapy of lung metastases of soft tissue sarcomas is 10 months [13]. These are the statistical tumor-biological facts on which we have to orient ourselves when we have to decide which treatments can influence the natural course of the disease. On the other hand, there are individual cases where a patient survives many years without any specific therapy. This should be held in mind when we consider the effectiveness of surgical therapy. For these reasons it seems to be without doubt that with this manner of treatment the median survival time as well as the 5-year survival time can be improved (table I).

It should be mentioned that the information regarding this differs considerably. Although a median survival time of between 12 and 36 months has been reported, the 5-year survival rate varies between 20 and 46%. The foundation for these different statements are in need of interpretation and are based on various disturbance factors which have to be known before the value of the therapeutic measures can be considered.

Differences in the survival time following surgical intervention of lung metastases of soft tissue sarcomas can be based on the location of the primary tumor, especially its tumor biology which is determined by the histological tumor type and tumor grading [9, 13].

Table I. Survival time following surgical therapy of pulmonary metastases from soft tissue sarcomas in adults

Author	Number of patients	5-Year survival rate	Median survival (months)
Turney [15]	25	46%	not given
McCormack [9]	202	35%	36
Creagan [2]	112	29%	18
Vogt-Moykopf [17]	28	23%	12
Putnam [11]	67	20%	24

There are also known behavioral differences in the various sarcomas, whereby it has to be taken into consideration whether the lung metastases appeared following a local recurrence which has been treated [16]. There are other factors besides the primary therapy which make a standardized and guarded assessment of the value of surgical therapy of metastasized soft tissue sarcomas very difficult if not impossible at this time. It has to remain open how much, if at all, other therapeutic measures, such as radio- or chemotherapy, as supplemental therapy to surgical intervention of lung metastases influence the final results. The results with systemic chemotherapy show that this effect should not be underestimated [1, 18]. The response rate for combination chemotherapy is, at a 40% rate of remission, considerable. The most effective single substance here are anthracyclines. Decisive for our consideration is that the median survival time of patients who respond to polychemotherapy equals those of patients treated by surgical resection of lung metastases of soft tissue sarcomas.

It has to be noted that there is a paucity of literature on the effectiveness of chemotherapy for patients with exclusive metastasizing of soft tissue sarcomas to the lung, so that a comparison with the surgically treated groups is limited. It should be mentioned that it is known through tests that the more favorable response of metastases of the lung to chemotherapy is during the limited disease stage, even in cases which were at first considered for surgical therapy [18]. No questioning of surgical therapy is intended with these remarks, but the importance of a precise limitation for its indication should be pointed out.

The objective is to determine the special criteria for an indication of surgical removal of metastases of soft tissue sarcoma in the adult.

The disease-free interval can be considered as an important criteria (table II). Patients with a disease-free interval of over 12 months from the time of primary surgery until the appearance of metastases to the lung profit by the surgical intervention compared to patients with a disease-free interval of less than 12 months. The survival time of untreated patients with a recurrence-free interval of over 12 month is less than that of patients who had surgical treatment of their lung metastases. The theory that the disease-free interval is only an expression of the therapy-independent aggression of the tumor cannot be substantiated, as shown in this retrospective analysis [8].

Another criterium in the guidelines of surgical therapy of metastases is the tumor doubling time (table III). The prognosis of patients with a tumor doubling time of under 40 days cannot generally be influenced by surgical therapy measures, whereas the median postoperative survival time of patients with a tumor doubling time of over 40 days is distinctively more favorable [2, 10–12].

Table II. Pulmonary metastases from soft tissue sarcomas in adults. Median survival following surgical therapy in relationship to the disease-free interval

Author	Number of patients	Median survival (months)	
		Interval < 12	Interval > 12
Huang [6]	50	23	25
Creagan [2]	112	12	24
Huth [7]	43	20	48 +
Roth [12]	67	10	30

Table III. Pulmonary metastases from soft tissue sarcomas in adults. Median survival following surgical therapy in relationship to tumor doubling time (TDT)

Author	Number of patients	Median survival (months)	
		TDT < 40 days	TDT > 40 days
Joseph [8]	113	12	24 +
Huang [6]	50	11	22
Huth [7]	43	7	20
Roth [12]	67	6	22

Besides the disease-free interval and tumor doubling time it is prognostically important whether a local recurrence has preceded the metastatic process in the lung. In these instances the chances of surgical
treatment of metastatic disease are extremely reduced [16]. Of question-
able influence for the prognosis is whether the completely removed lung
metastasis is a solitary or singular, bi- or unilateral manifestation [2, 14].
Seemingly, the histological tumor type is of secondary importance [10],
but it should be considered here that only certain soft tissue sarcomas
metastasize primarily to the lung [16] and that they dominate in the corresponding statistics so much that, based on the relatively few cases,
judgement errors are possible.

The factors outlined may consequently explain some of the differences in the prognostic statements of surgically treated patients with
lung metastases of soft tissue sarcoma. Additionally, it is interesting to
point out a phenomenon, namely that, as seen over the years, the 5-year
curative rate of surgically treated patients has declined (table I). This
could indicate that lately the indications for surgical intervention have
been interpreted far too generously. The above-mentioned factors
should be considered closely in the decisions for surgical therapy of lung
metastases. Possibly preoperative chemotherapy can influence the survival time of patients with an unfavorable prognosis [7].

The experiences gained in the treatment of metastases of the lung
at the University of California should be incorporated into our treatment plan. It was shown that even in cases of unfavorable prognosis
patients who responded to preoperative chemotherapy had a much
higher survival time than expected on the basis of historical studies. Besides the possibility of an improved estimation of the tumor growth
rate, preoperative chemotherapy offers an advantage in recognizing
cytostatic-sensitive tumors, and therefore it is easier to plan an appropriate postoperative chemotherapy. A deterioration of the prognosis
due to delay of surgical treatment does not have any influence on the
course of the disease in any case, as some analyses have shown [6].

In conclusion, it can be stated that the surgical removal of lung
metastases of soft tissue sarcomas in adults has its importance and legi-
timacy. The entire curative effect should not be overestimated. It also
has to be considered that not every pulmonary finding in patients with
anamnestically-known soft tissue sarcoma necessarily indicates metastases (table IV). Favorable conditions for effective surgical therapy of
lung metastases is a prolonged disease-free interval following the prim-

Table IV. Portion of pulmonary metastases in patients with soft tissue sarcomas showing 'round lesions' on chest X-ray

Author	Number of patients	Number of patients with metastases
Johnson [19]	24	20/24 (83%)
Flye [4]	41	35/41 (85%)

ary tumor surgery and a relatively slow tumor doubling rate of the lung metastases. Experience has shown that a favorable response to preoperative chemotherapy seems to be of superior prognostic importance and should therefore be included in all future multimodal therapy plans.

References

1 Blum, R. H.; Corson, J. M. et al.: Successful treatment of metastatic sarcomas with cyclophosphamide, adriamycin and DTIC (CAD). Cancer *46:* 1722–1726 (1980).

2 Creagan, E. T.; Fleming, T. R.; Edmonson, J. H.; Pairolero, P.: Pulmonary resection for metastatic monosteogenic sarcoma. Cancer *44:* 1908–1912 (1979).

3 Feldman, Ph. S.; Kyriakos, M.: Pulmonary resection for metastatic sarcoma. J. thorac. cardiovasc. Surg. *64:* 784–799 (1972).

4 Flye, M. W.; Woltering, G.; Rosenberg, S. A.: Aggressive pulmonary resection for metastatic osteogenic and soft tissue sarcomas. Ann. thor. Surg. *37:* 123–127 (1984).

5 Fuchs, R.; Esterhausen, M.; Makoski, H.-B.; Andrian-Werberg, H., Freiherr von: Therapie der Weichteilsarkome. Dt. med. Wschr. *111:* 710–713 (1986).

6 Huang, M. N.; Edgerton, F.; Takita, H. et al.: Lung resection for metastatic sarcoma. Am. J. Surg. *135:* 804–806 (1978).

7 Huth, J. F.; Holmes, E. C.; Vernon, S. E. et al.: Pulmonary resection for metastatic sarcoma. Am. J. Surg. *140:* 9–16 (1980).

8 Joseph, W. L.; Morton, D. L.; Adkins, P. C.: Prognostic significance of tumor doubling time in evaluating operability in pulmonary metastatic disease. J. thorac. cardiovasc. Surg. *61:* 23–32 (1971).

9 McCormack, P. M.; Martini, N.: The changing role of surgery for pulmonary metastases. Ann. thor. Surg. *28:* 139–145 (1979).

10 Morrow, Ch. E.; Vassilopoulos, P. P.; Grage, Th. B.: Surgical resection for metastatic neoplasms of the lung: experience at the University of Minnesota Hospitals. Cancer *45:* 2981–2985 (1980).

11 Putnam, J. B.; Roth, J. A.; Wesley, M. et al.: Analysis of prognostic factors in patients undergoing resection of pulmonary metastases from soft tissue sarcomas. J. thorac. cardiovasc. Surg. *87:* 260–268 (1984).

12 Roth, J. A.; Putnam, J. B.; Wesley, M. N.; Rosenberg, St. A.: Differing determinants of prognosis following resection of pulmonary metastases from osteogenic and soft tissue sarcoma patients. Cancer *55:* 1361–1366 (1985).

13 Shieber, W.; Graham, P.: An experience with sarcomas of the soft tissue in adults. Surgery *52:* 295–299 (1962).

14 Takita, H.; Merrin, C.; Didolkar, M. S. et al.: The surgical management of multiple lung metastases. Ann. thor. Surg. *24:* 359–364 (1977).

15 Turney, St. Z.; Haight, C.; Arbor, A.: Pulmonary resection for metastatic neoplasms. J. thorac. cardiovasc. Surg. *61:* 784–794 (1971).

16 Vezeridis, M. P.; Moore, R.; Karakousis, C. P.: Metastatic patterns in soft-tissue sarcomas. Arch. Surg. *118:* 915–918 (1983).

17 Vogt-Moykopf, I.; Toomes, H.; Paul, K.; Abel, U.: Die chirurgische Therapie der Lungenmetastasen: Indikation, Technik, Ergebnisse. Arch. klin. Chir. *361:* 533–537 (1983).

18 Yap, B.-S.; Rasmussen, S. L.; Burgess, M. A. et al.: Prognostic factors in adults with advanced soft tissue sarcomas. ASCO Abstracts C-608: 473 (1980).

19 Johnson, H.; Fantone, J.; Flye, W. H.: Histological evaluation of the nodules resected in the treatment of pulmonary metastatic disease. J. Surg. Oncol. *21:* 1–4 (1982).

Prof. Dr. med. P. Schlag, Leiter der Sektion für chirurgische Onkologie,
Chirurgische Universitätsklinik, Im Neuenheimer Feld 110,
D-6900 Heidelberg 1 (FRG)